"Dr. Serin has cracked the code o[   ] treatment available to everyone. I can't go to sleep because of their st[   ] gives you and them a clear, easy-to-use process for reducing stress and anxiety nearly instantly. If you want to flip the switch on stress, get a better night of sleep and take control of stress once and for all, read this book today. This is my new go-to book on stress for all my patients."

—MICHAEL BREUS, PHD

Author of *The Power of When* and *The Sleep Doctor's Diet Plan*, and Member of the clinical advisory board for *The Dr. Oz Show*

"Dr. Amy Serin is a stand-out figure in leading-edge Neuropsychology. She takes mind/body work to a new level with *The Stress Switch*. In it, she describes with elegant detail an advanced understanding of the patterns of dysregulation stress causes in our nervous system. She rightly concludes that both past trauma and the current world of worry have greatly changed our collective inner worlds for the worse. More importantly, she explains step-by-step methods she has discovered to rapidly short-circuit stress responses and take your life back. Her work as an author, clinician and inventor in the field of Neuropsychology is groundbreaking. She explains how these unhealthy stress response patters have been locked in to our brain circuit wiring. Her work can help you regain control through renewed understanding of the patterns that need to be changed, while giving you the tools to rapidly make these changes."

—ROBERT D. SHEELER, MD

Associate Professor Emeritus, Mayo Medical School, Former editor, *Mayo Clinic Health Letter*, and Former chair, Mayo Foundation Neuropsychiatric Medicine Task Force

"*The Stress Switch* is a breakthrough on many levels. Dr. Serin's deep clinical background and extensive expertise in Neuropsychology have given her unique insights into what is wrong with the modern world. Stress consumes many of us and eats away at the foundations of our relationships, our work, and our happiness. Dr. Serin explains the foundations of this problem in an approachable way that can be understood by anyone with interest in making a change for the better. In my work with executives, complex patients, adolescents and young children I find that stress is a key element that underlies many of the conditions they suffer from. Dr. Serin makes it clear that stress is not your fault. It is the result of faulty wiring of our brain pathways and false interpretations that lock the stress switch in the ON position. The good news is that, with the insights and understandings she offers, it is possible to rapidly flip the stress switch back to the OFF position. As her work is embraced it will be a large step toward healing and health. I intend to recommend her book to all my patients."

—ANGELA O'NEIL, MD
Former Assistant Professor and Assistant Dean, Mayo Medical School

"Dr. Serin literally saved my life. I wouldn't be the man I am today without her, and I am forever grateful. When I asked a friend years ago for a reference to help me with my panic and overwhelming stress after I went to several doctors who didn't help, he told me, 'Go to Dr. Serin. Don't go anywhere else. And do whatever she says because it will change your life.' When I remember that moment, I thank God I listened. I think everyone's lives could improve from following the advice in this book."

—RON F., 44
Former patient, the Serin Center clinics

The Stress Switch

Dr. Amy Serin

SIMPLY
GOOD PRESS
EST. 2012

THE
STRESS
SWITCH

THE TRUTH ABOUT STRESS AND HOW TO SHORT-CIRCUIT IT

DR. AMY SERIN

SIMPLY GOOD PRESS / MONTCLAIR

Published by Simply Good Press, Montclair, New Jersey.
www.simplygoodpress.com
Printed in the United States of America.
© 2019 by Amy Serin.

The author of this book does not dispense medical advice or prescribe the use of any technique, either directly or indirectly, as a form of treatment for physical, emotional, or medical problems, without the advice of a physician. The author's intent is only to offer information of a general nature to help you in your quest for emotional, physical, and spiritual well-being. In the event you use any of the information in this book, the author and the publisher assume no responsibility for your actions.

For permissions requests, speaking inquiries, and bulk-order purchase options, visit www.amyserin.com.

Cover designed by Scott C. Leuthold
Interior designed by Erika Cole Gillette

Library of Congress Control Number: 2019935725

ISBN-13: 978-1-7326-5215-6 (paper)
ISBN-13: 978-1-7326-5216-3 (.mobi)

To the love, joy, and light that is the essence of your true nature. May it help you uncover what is real.
And to my beloved sons, Christopher and Connor.

CONTENTS

PREFACE

I've been gifted with the opportunity to have helped heal thousands of people in my twelve years of clinical neuropsychology practice and there is one unwavering truth that I have learned. When you resolve trauma, reduce stress, and heal, what lies beneath the layers of soot of suffering is pure beauty. When a person uncovers this, love and kindness towards the self and towards others is the only thing left. It is our true essence. Creativity flows, and a sense of connection with all things instantly dissipate the problematic ego. The result is higher consciousness, greater intention of action, and the loss of fear. This state of being is so beautiful and attainable that I resolved to make it my life's work to reduce suffering so that humanity can re-emerge into this state on a broad scale.

And this is a crucial goal to achieve, because we are suffering! As individuals and a collective we are suffering! Despite my knowledge and training, I'm certainly not immune from the human condition; I suffer myself when I get bogged down in the complexity of life and the stories I tell myself about it. Coupled with a human nervous system that does what it wants without my conscious control, I'm unable to attain the feeling states I want in certain moments. But to the extent that I practice what I preach, I am able to be calm and centered enough to carry forward with purpose so that others can benefit. And as you'll learn in this book, when we misunderstand the stress switch and how it operates within us, we use inefficient, outdated strategies without results. Then we beat ourselves up for our behavior and lack of control, and the cycle repeats.

We believe the inaccuracies of a medical system that tells us our problems are lifelong and can only be managed with marginal success. We helplessly watch our loved ones suffer and assume their suffering will be lifelong too, because we are without an understanding of how we can effectively remove their suffering and prevent an unraveling of the spirit or post-traumatic stress disorder (PTSD). And we hurt others and perpetuate the problem when we don't take care of ourselves.

But there is hope. In an effort to prevent and heal the global PTSD epidemic, I discovered that a trusted technology—one which has been used in therapeutic modalities for over thirty years—could be isolated and delivered using wearable devices beyond a clinical setting to dim down the stress switch in real time. Based on a body of scientific research and over two dozen research studies and scientific presentations, my company developed wearable devices to deliver the technology called *TouchPoints,* and our technology has been shown to reduce stress by sixty-two percent in thirty seconds, stabilize cortisol faster after stress than a control group, produce profound changes on electroencephalograms of children and adults, help people fall asleep faster, and even reduce physical pain. In my Serin Center clinics in Arizona, we use TouchPoints in conjunction with eye movement desensitization and reprocessing (EMDR therapy) (a psychotherapy treatment that helps heal the symptoms resulting from traumatic life experiences), neurofeedback (mapping real-time electroencephalogram brain function and using operant conditioning to regulate it), neuromodulation, and integrative care, and we are able to do better than help people cope with stress and suffering and transform people's lives.

When I set out to develop the technology that became TouchPoints, I never dreamed that I would uncover the truths I'm sharing with you in this book. I had no idea that my own ideas about stress were unrefined and misguided at times, or that thirty seconds with the devices we were creating could spontaneously generate positive thinking and a feeling of well-being without conscious effort, nor did I imagine that a disturbing memory of a stressful event could be almost neutralized and would never re-occur with the same

"Oh no!" reaction again. You see, I was a product of my doctoral training, and I had accepted the status quo like so many other researchers and doctors—until I had the courage to innovate beyond what I was taught. For a few years, I had given my patients prescriptions for stress management and believed they couldn't heal from certain diagnoses. I'm happy to say that I've evolved beyond this limited thinking and I'm so excited to share this with you.

With this book, my goal is to tell the truth about stress and suffering, clear up misguided assumptions and incomplete information for you, and explain why you can't outwit stress. You aren't flawed for not being in control of your stress. You've been misguided by a system that doesn't understand what we are really dealing with. You've been duped into overestimating how consciousness and chemicals can affect the brain, because the entire world is missing the simplicity of how the brain and body really work. The result is that we've overlooked the possible cure. Until now. Please join me in my quest to help you personally achieve a more calm, centered, intentional life so that you can uncover your own inner light and live into your best life. And please believe me when I tell you that you can have more than you ever imagined.

—AMY SERIN, PhD

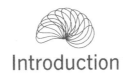

Introduction

STRESSED OUT!

"75% of adults reported experiencing moderate to high levels of stress in the past month and nearly half reported that their stress has increased in the past year."
—The American Psychological Association 2009 Stress Survey[1]

"Research shows for the first time that the effects of psychological stress on the body's ability to regulate inflammation can promote the development and progression of disease."
—Carnegie Mellon University research study[2]

"Stress is a top health concern for U.S. teens between 9th and 12th grade. Psychologists say that if they don't learn healthy ways to manage that stress now, it could have serious long-term health implications."
—The American Psychological Association[3]

You lie awake at night worrying, worrying some more, worrying that you're worrying too much, and then worrying that you'll never be able to stop worrying. Even if you're not a worrier, stress can hit you like a wave multiple times daily, and follow you into your sleep at night. It's like the movie *Groundhog Day*—lather, rinse, repeat the next night, and wake up every morning beating yourself up for being unable to fight this *thing* that has overtaken your life for so long. This thing called stress.

We're not just *stressed* here in America. We are *so* stressed that our nervous systems respond to everyday events as if we're living in the war zone of a third-world country, scrounging to feed our families while ducking under a continuous hail of bullets. Even though we aren't under threat, our nervous systems act as though we are. We could be peacefully arriving five minutes late to events, or calmly returning a phone call later if we don't answer when it rings, or reminding our brain that it's making mountains out of molehills as we fret over things that really aren't a big deal. But most of the time we don't. Why?

Today's news headlines reveal that as a society we are all too familiar with the signs and symptoms of stress—insomnia, weight gain, decreased attention span, anxiety, depression, heart disease, digestive disorders, and more.

Our unchecked stress levels are literally waging a war against our minds, bodies, lives, families, and communities. Individual stress merges into a collective state of worry and the result is a global crisis of stress. This is because when stress runs willy-nilly through our bodies like a bull in a china shop, it puts us in a chronic, reactionary state. When we're no longer living life, but just reacting to it, our constant state of alert negatively impacts the people around us, too.

In today's world, our nervous system's natural, adrenaline-fueled, evolutionary fight-or-flight responses are overused and overactive. Fight-or-flight normally happens when your nervous system senses a threat to your life, overrides your thinking brain, and decides whether your greatest chances of survival will come from putting up your dukes and fighting the threat or from running away from it. Biologically, a fight-or-flight response is only supposed to happen in life-or-death situations.

Most of us are in a chronic state of stress that fluctuates at levels high enough to cause our nervous systems to think we're in mortal danger. Take a moment to think about how this is affecting your life and relationships with your partner, your children, your coworkers, and your community. When you snap at others, make impulsive decisions, slam doors, hang up the phone in frustration, yell at your children or partner, binge on "comfort food" (or comfort adult beverages), you can thank stress. It's normal to have stressful moments, but for many of us, stress has become a chronic reactionary state. Living in this type of biological "code red" situation affects your highest potential in life and what you're capable of achieving personally and professionally.

Our stress doesn't operate in a vacuum, either. Rather, one person's stress acts like toxic mercury released into a pond. Ripple by ripple, the toxin spreads. It touches everyone we encounter in this state. We pollute their chances of being calm and happy, because they pick up on our stress—and our behaviors activate their own stress systems.

Now, think about that on a national scale. Our collective stress condition as a country affects how we deal with each other and with the world as a whole. Seen this way, stress escalates from a personal problem to a global one. Stress is no longer just your problem to deal with—it's everyone's problem. The stress of the politicians on the news, your co-workers, and your loved ones all affect you, and vice versa. Do you really want to change the world? When you're in survival mode, you may be changing it indeed, but not for the better. Ouch.

It may seem especially surprising that the problem of stress appears unsolvable, given the plethora of stress management programs available to the general public, along with rampant articles and books on the topic of managing stress. To be clear, this book will not regurgitate the old strategies. My aims here are to reveal the shocking truths behind stress—what causes it, the great dangers of letting it run amok, and why the current programs to combat it have categorically failed—and most importantly, to offer a total paradigm shift around how you understand and deal with stress.

The biggest question is, how on Earth did this happen? Here in the U.S., people live generally good lives. For the most part we have freedom, safety, shelter, food, water, and comfort to spare. Why, then, aren't our rates of personal fulfillment and health outcomes better? Why is stress torpedoing our happiness? Why aren't people living better lives? How is it that somebody in a third-world country who makes $50 a month is happier and less stressed than we are? What are we *not getting* about stress and what to do about it?

The answer may begin with the fact that our culture, including our medical community, has a problem with the way we view stress. We're not looking at it or talking about it correctly. And how are you supposed to solve a problem you don't fully understand?

We've somehow decided that stress is a normal part of life—totally inevitable and unavoidable. So we add stress management as an item on our things-to-do list. Our most popular stress "solutions" actually add more of the stuff that stresses us out to our plates. There's the time investment (from treatment), money investment (often at an exorbitant level for treatment fail after treatment fail), and the anxiety that comes from all the added to-dos on your list to manage stress. It's no wonder that the result is you're still stressed.

In our modern, overly scheduled lives, we struggle for a rigorous daily regimen of proper, socially approved stress relief: get enough sleep so you can get up early to meditate, go to yoga, go to the gym, go outdoors into the sunshine, schedule a massage, schedule a spa day, schedule acupuncture, schedule a vacation—squeeze it all in so you're not stressed! And that's just for you. If you're a parent, you've been told to make sure the children meditate, go to yoga, exercise, play with their peers, play sports, take music lessons, eat a perfect diet, strive to be well-rounded and well-adjusted, and see a counselor if they're not playing well with others.... all in the name of stress management. God forbid we—or our children—miss a beat; Rome would surely fall. Stress management can be stressful, can't it?

We're missing the point. We've designed our lives around accommodating something that we've been made to believe is a chronic, lifelong, incurable condition. If the information you're working from is that stress has no solution, your focus becomes solely on dealing with it. Managing it. Coping with it. Trying to think our way out of it, or through it. Those are inadequate options because consciousness is not as strong as the stress system.

But what if I told you that excess stress was *not* a chronic, permanent condition to be managed, but rather that it has a switch that can be turned on—often without your awareness—and that it can be turned off almost instantaneously, too? A switch like this could regulate the stress response in moments when it's not necessary—effectively short-circuiting the tripwires that cause stress to be turned on excessively? And what if I told you that more often than not, the "stress switch" does turn on unnecessarily, and that our society has it wrong when they insist that the switch needs to stay on, and you'll just need to accept it? If you knew that stress has a switch that YOU have the power to turn on and off, but not in the ways that you've been told—how would that change how you manage stress?

This audacity comes primarily from my work as a neuropsychologist in my Serin Center clinics, helping to rewrite my patients' stress stories, and the stress stories their children have inherited from them—that stress is unavoidable, chronic, and for many, an utterly hopeless battle. As a mom myself, these stories, incorrect beliefs about stress, and inefficient methods to try to treat stress fuel my mission. Here is the bottom line. I do not want my children to suffer. No parent does. I have looked directly into the face of stress and understood the enemy, and I refuse to let my children suffer from its crippling effects. I will not let it cast its dark shadow over our lives.

I don't want you or your children to succumb to this enemy either. With this book I'm sharing my purpose and my life's work with you because I need your help. Changing a national paradigm around the nature of stress and how to cure it is no small mission. But I am offering up solutions, and I'd like you to join me.

Joining this mission begins with your personal choice to understand the true nature of stress. Watch and learn as I pull back the curtain on the lies we've been told about it. Then, together, we can take an honest look at how stress acts like mercury in a pond, poisoning everything in our body's ecosystem from sleep to empathy, and influencing us to lose our tempers and become selfish. Finally, armed with these new (often shocking) truths about stress, you'll be ready for rewiring so you can serve as an example for your family, your community, and ultimately our nation and the world. In the new paradigm, where the stress switch is short-circuited instead of simply managed, you will live a life of your greatest good and highest potential rather than a life of mere survival, doing daily battle with an invisible, seemingly indestructible enemy.

If this is a far more serious conversation about stress than you're used to, it's because that's how serious the future implications are if we continue down this path. We are a great nation full of good-hearted people who each possess infinite potential to achieve remarkable things and impact the world in positive ways. But in order to be successful, we must remove this thing called stress that is robbing us of our future in every moment we let it. That is my mission for this book and beyond. I hope you will read on, and join me.

"If you saw Atlas, the giant who holds the world on his shoulders, if you saw that he stood, blood running down his chest, his knees buckling, his arms trembling but still trying to hold the world aloft with the last of his strength, and the greater his effort the heavier the world bore down upon his shoulders—what would you tell him?"
-Ayn Rand, *Atlas Shrugged*

Carrying all that weight weakens your ability to do anything else. I'd tell Atlas to set it down. And P.S. regarding stress, I'm pretty sure Atlas is a woman.

Part I: Do No Harm

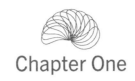

Chapter One

THE ULTIMATE DISRUPTER

Breathe easy. There are neurological reasons why you can't 'outwit' stress as you've been trying. You aren't flawed for not being able to control it. You are human. It's time to honor the neurological basis of your humanity and move forward.

Nervous System 101

Understanding stress starts with understanding its habitat, the nervous system. If you already have this knowledge of Nervous System 101, I invite you to please skip forward to the next section of this chapter.

For the rest of you, this anatomy overview is essential to understanding how the nervous system works, how stress sets it off, and why setting it off is largely outside of your control. This will also explain why stress isn't something that can simply be outwitted by attempts at logical thinking. In other words, if you are feeling defeated because you haven't been able to think away that stress you've been carrying around, go easy on yourself. It's not your fault.

Let's take a tour of the house where your stress lives. Your nervous system is a collection of nerves and specialized cells called neurons, which transmit signals between the different parts of the body. The nervous system has two parts: the **central nervous system** and the **peripheral nervous system**. The only difference between central nerves and peripheral nerves is their location in the body. The central nervous system includes the nerves, brain, and spinal cord, and it's contained in the skull and vertebral canal of the spine. All the nerves in the body outside of those in the skull and spine are part of the peripheral nervous system.

The nerves in your body are classified a different way as well— according to what kinds of functions they control—into the involuntary and voluntary nervous systems. The **involuntary nervous system** is also called your **autonomic nervous system**, with "auto" here meaning self-directed. The **voluntary nervous system** is correspondingly called your **somatic nervous system**, which controls the things you're aware of and can influence conscious actions such as moving your arms and legs. Both the central and peripheral nervous systems have voluntary and involuntary parts.

The involuntary, or somatic, nervous system regulates the unconscious processes in the body such as breathing, heart rate, and metabolic processes like carb, sugar and fat cell breakdown; it accomplishes this regulation by sending signals from the body to the brain or the brain to the body. So, if you get too hot, your involuntary nervous system increases the blood circulation to your skin and makes you sweat more. And when you're stressed, your breathing changes without your awareness.

To define the nervous system into even more specific categories, the involuntary nervous system is made up of the **sympathetic nervous system**, also known as your fight-or-flight nervous system, and the **parasympathetic nervous system,** which is the system devoted to relaxation.

At its evolutionary roots, your sympathetic nervous system exists to prepare you for emergencies, and to do so, it shuts down all functions that aren't necessary for a quick escape or fight in a life-or-death situation. We call this state **sympathetically activated**. The sympathetic system prepares you for physical and mental activity, makes your heart beat faster, opens up airways so you can breathe deeper, and inhibits body functions that are not essential in emergency situations.

One the other hand, the parasympathetic system is responsible for all those biological housekeeping functions you enjoy when you're peacefully at rest, like digesting food and other metabolic processes your body needs to live. If you need a memory trick, think "stressed out sympathetic" and "peaceful parasympathetic."

The sympathetic and parasympathetic nervous systems are connected and can work simultaneously, but current medical knowledge suggests that when the sympathetic nervous system is active, the parasympathetic nervous system is inactive, and vice versa. Think of it like this—if your fight-or-flight is on, your biological housekeeping is off, even though they're still working in conjunction with each other.

Really let that one sink in, because we're going to take a hard look at its ramifications: when you are sympathetically activated in order to stay alive in an urgent moment, all kinds of important stuff that keeps you alive in all the other moments *stops working.*

Salience Network

Within the central nervous system is a key brain network responsible for deciding what to do based on what is going on inside and outside of your body. This **salience network** decides what is important (salient) and signals a shift in attentional states to what is important. Without your conscious awareness, it also can flip the switch of the sympathetic nervous system based on what it senses. Your salience network is constantly deciding, "Based on the sensory information coming in right now, should I be internally focused or externally focused? Am I going to be stressed or calm?"

This large-scale network is anchored in regions of the brain called the anterior insula and dorsal anterior cingulate cortex, and is made up of three key structures: the amygdala, the ventral striatum, and the substantia nigra/ventral tegmental area.[4] Now, I don't expect you to know what those areas of the brain do, but you've probably heard of the amygdala—the almond-shaped structure that is directly responsible for setting off the fight-or-flight response. What most people ignore when discussing the amygdala is how, when, and based on what information it makes the decision to turn the stress response on or off. The key lies with the other structures in the salience network: they sense and integrate information into signals that are sent to the amygdala, and then the amygdala provides feedback.

The salience network contributes to a variety of brain functions, including communication, social behavior, and self-awareness, by integrating sensory, emotional, and cognitive information. And this is why you should rethink what you think you know about stress and how much control you think you have over it. **The salience network's job is to do its thing without your awareness.** See, awareness (consciousness) is inefficient, so your brain is adept at only bringing your attention to things that it has learned you need to think about. And when you are in fight-or-flight, thinking about what you should do can be a deadly waste of time because consciousness is slow compared with knee-jerk reactions. So the salience network senses something dangerous, integrates it without your awareness, turns on the stress switch, and a cascade of physical changes inflames your body, shutting down all non-essential functions.

And what is non-essential for survival in the moment when your brain is signaling a threat? Basically every function that separates humans from animals! Social communication, self-awareness, and the ability to think through consequences all shut down in stress mode, basically turning you into a ball of reactivity and impulse. Ever said something you didn't mean out of anger during a fight with your partner? Ever made a wrong turn when you were in a hurry even though you knew the way to your destination? Ever screamed when you saw a bug and felt embarrassed in a public place? Ever felt so afraid to do something that you panicked, even though the fear was imagined? You have your salience network, sympathetic nervous system, and survival mechanisms to thank for that, and you're not alone.

In contrast, when your stress switch is off, you are calm, focused, able to communicate, empathetic to others around you, and also able to think clearly. If you've left work to take a break and suddenly strategic answers to a problem present themselves, if you've found yourself to be more engaged with people after a yoga class or a nice relaxing experience, you can understand how being in this mode creates much more desirable behavior and clear thinking.

Now what is great about the salience network is that it's doing a lot of good things for you. Take a moment and tune in to your environment right now. There might be background noise you haven't noticed. There may be an air conditioner on, cars whizzing by on the street outside, or maybe people talking in the next room. Without your awareness, your salience network senses and integrates these things along with any pain sensations and decides—based on a complex matrix of biological programming, past experiences, and the current state of your brain and body—what it's going to bring to your attention. Wherever you are and whatever you're doing, your salience network acts like an unconscious flight control radar that tracks everything it senses in the air. Your salience network senses and records all the sights, sounds, smells, tastes, and tactile sensations your body is receiving and decides what to do with the information.

Fortunately, you're not aware of this ever-present, finely tuned radar that's constantly processing everything coming in through your bodily senses. And why does it do this without your awareness? Well, if you had to think every second about how your pants felt on your legs, it would monopolize so much of your cognitive brainpower that you wouldn't be able to function!

Right now, your salience network is helping you tune everything else out so you can focus and comprehend the words you're reading on this page, instead of keying in on every single sensory stimulus around you. The salience network is integrating all that sensory information from the outside AND it's also integrating information from the inside of your body. In mere milliseconds, this critical neurological network takes in all that information and decides what to do with your attention and how to adjust your stress switch, whether that means turning the switch completely on, completely off, or adjusting it somewhere in between. In fact, your stress switch operates like a dimmer switch. Your salience network uses input from your senses to turn your stress switch on, and additionally, how much to turn it *up*. Your salience network has its metaphorical finger on your stress switch at all times, assessing sensory information as it comes in, and turning the switch up or down, on or off, in response.

Maria

I had a seventeen-year-old patient named Maria who was very anxious, extremely high-achieving, and perfectionistic. Her mother often entered the house, saw that a chore wasn't done to her liking, and launched into a full-on fit.

Looking for a way to diffuse the situation, Maria would ask, "What exactly would you like me to do? What didn't I do correctly?"

Her mom would respond, "Well, you should know!" and the tirade would continue.

This is a very twisted cycle for a high-achieving, perfectionist people-pleaser like my patient to be put through time and time again. Imagine if every time you cleaned your house, right on cue, a tornado would tear through, undoing all the order you just created.

Every time tornado mom's stress switch was on, she would have these fits, and Maria's stress switch would turn on as well. Merely thinking about these episodes locked Maria's neck muscles so badly that she had her massage therapist and chiropractor on speed dial as her only forms of (temporary) relief. Here was a young girl without any structural or functional physical abnormality that would be causing muscle tension and pain. This was purely a stress reaction.

We worked with Maria in a variety of ways, all aimed at stopping her nervous system from activating and creating her physical stress reaction just from thinking about her mother and this traumatic physical situation she has lived with her entire life. There was a lot to reverse here, including teaching her how to not take it personally.

Working from the standpoint of the nervous system, we focused on getting Maria's salience network to stop turning on the stress switch whenever she thought of her mom or whenever her mom entered as the tornado.

Like so many of my patients and others caught in these cycles of stress, Maria felt like she had tried it all by time she came to the Serin Center clinics. In addition to the neck tension and shoulder problems, she also had migraines and was on some pretty heavy medication.

After eight sessions of therapy at my clinic, Maria's migraines remitted by about ninety percent, and her visits to the other doctors are fewer and farther between. And we're not done yet....

Internal Fire Alarm

Say you're at a corporate board meeting and the actual building fire alarm goes off. Suddenly, the quarterly financials no longer matter because everyone is reacting to the alarm, grabbing their things, and evacuating the building. In the case of the real external fire alarm and also in your own internal stress alarm, nothing executive is happening in the brain either.

When deciding whether or not to flip the stress switch, your nervous system has an internal fire alarm built into it, and it's your salience network's job to decide how sensitive that alarm is. The better the job your salience network is doing, the more it will take to set off your fire alarm as you go about daily life. However, some of us have sensitive trip-wires. For instance, it takes very little to set off gifted and autistic individuals with sensory integration disorders. These individuals have a salience network that is not discriminating appropriately, leaving them with a sensitive internal switch that sets off their stress too often when the lights are a little bright, the temperature shifts, someone talks too loudly, etc.

Even for those of us whose salience networks are doing a pretty good job, a loud boom, the sight of a snake, a disappointed look on a loved one's face, and many other triggers based on your experiences and fears can cause your salience network to flick on your stress switch and activate your sympathetic nervous system in just milliseconds, launching you into an instant state of nervous system reactivity to the trigger. There, with your stress switch on, and without awareness, your heart begins pounding, your mind starts racing, you start breathing shallowly, and all aspects of brain and body function that are non-essential for survival take a back seat to impulsive reactivity.

When partners are arguing, it's important to determine to what degree the stress switch is on. When one person's switch is fully on but the other's is not, sometimes the calm partner can help turn the other's stress switch down so they can have a productive conversation. But (and this is the number one rule in couple's therapy) if both partner's stress switches are on, neither will be rational or calm, and any conversation might end up contentious and damaging to the relationship.

In their "Love Lab," famous couples' therapists Drs. John and Julie Gottman observe couples going about daily life activities such as eating breakfast and having typical conversations. They also observe couples discussing difficult topics. The Gottmans use technology to measure nervous system reactivity and biomarkers of stress in real-time. They realized that couples could appear calm on the outside at times when their stress switches were actually activated. Many couples reported feeling fine during a conversation with their partners, but their heart rates would be racing, and their blood pressure would be skyrocketing. Their stress switches were on and they didn't even know it. Why is this important? By measuring the stress response, the Gottmans can more accurately predict who is going to get divorced or be perpetually unhappy in their relationships.

One of the Gottmans' contributions to our field is teaching couples that when things get heated, and one or both partner's stress switches move to the on position, they need to go to their separate corners, self-soothe, and then come back to problem solve together when they are calm. That's easier said than done, because it hinges on accurate self-assessment as to whether your stress switch is on or off. When one or both members of the couple mistakenly thinks they're soothed enough to re-engage, they may still be reactive and say things they don't mean.

Psychologists have distinguished two distinct modes of behavior, called "minds," or "brains," to help identify this shift from the deliberate, rational action that is possible when we are calm to the impulsive and irrational behavior we experience when we are stressed. They label the rational mode the "**executive brain**," and the more primitive, irrational mode the "**lizard brain**." When you are stressed out, your executive brain—which is thoughtful, rational, compassionate, and reasonable—is essentially shut down. And the lizard brain—which is impulsive, reactive, and irrational—takes over. When you're stressed, your lizard brain is way more powerful than your executive brain. This is great news for survival, but not such great news when you need your reasoning skills to recognize that your stress is unwarranted, or to control your reactive behavior. The higher your stress switch goes, the less power your executive brain has and the more your lizard brain takes control. Stress switch on means lizard brain on and executive brain off!

Before we move on, it's important to review one more time how the salience network, stress, and the stress switch work together. Let's walk through the sequence step by step—although keep in mind that all these steps happen in milliseconds of real time!

Something stressful happens. For example, you step on a splinter, receive an IRS notice in the mail, have a stressful thought about something that happened at work, or a fire alarm goes off in your apartment building.

First, sensory input about the event travels from sensory organs such as your skin, eyes, or ears to your brain. In the case of a thought, information travels through your brain's internal neural networks.

Next, your salience network assesses the information and decides how much to turn up your stress switch, and how quickly to move it from low to high, based on what else is happening in your environment and in your body. For instance, while a fire alarm will set the switch immediately to high, a mildly disturbing thought might slowly inch the switch from off to low.

Before you are even aware of it, your stress switch is on, and a chain reaction of chemical and physical changes is taking place in your body according to where the switch has been turned.

Now, you are in some degree of sympathetic activation, and your executive brain is compromised to a corresponding degree. The higher your stress switch is turned on, the harder it will be to turn it down and off. What's more, the journey back to off is not a 1:1 ratio, meaning that bringing your stress switch it back down again will take more than the few seconds it took that fire alarm to send it up.

You can't easily "think" your stress switch down once it has been activated by your salience network, which brings us to our next topic of discussion: how your brain and body are *actually* connected.

Mind/Body Neurology

Now that you've learned the basics of how the salience network controls the switch between stressed and calm states, let's look at how it connects to your mind. Here, and from now on, I'm using the word "mind" to refer to your consciousness, something that, historically speaking, hasn't always been closely associated with the concrete biology of the body.

The French philosopher Rene Descartes (1596-1650) argued that the mind and the body are completely separate entities, and that one can exist separately from the other.[5] Even today, hundreds of years and significant scientific advances later, a good number of laypeople and even medical professionals treat the mind and body as completely separate things. Descartes' famous statement, *Cogito ergo sum*, translates to "I think, therefore I am," meaning that there is a consciousness that can doubt or question things. As humans, we can think about our thoughts, and this consciousness also observes the body, which is separate from the mind.

However, having studied neuroscience and healed thousands of people over the last decade, what is apparent to me is that this "mind" isn't a detached observer. The mind's observations are only possible based on what the salience network selects for attention. It's all connected and integrated, and we need to re-attach what has been literally dismembered in our construct of how we think everything works. Ironically, some of the most compelling proof of integration can be found in medicine. One example is phantom limb pain, in which, after an amputation, an individual still experiences physical sensations of pain—as if their arm or leg is still attached to their body. If untreated, these signals can continue being transmitted to the brain not just directly after the amputation, but for the remainder of the person's life. Why? Because the experience of pain happens in your brain, not in your leg. So while the original pain was caused by a real physical injury that sent a signal (or set of signals) to your nervous system, later, the memory networks can recreate the signal that past pain initiated, by memory. So when an associational memory, habit, or other trigger causes the brain to recreate that original signal, the individual feels pain in a limb that is no longer there. The same process occurs for both physical and emotional pain, too. That's why a sound or smell that triggers a memory of a traumatic event can send an abuse survivor into fight-or-flight mode. The brain works on habits and shortcuts, so if you have felt pain once, you are more likely to feel it again, because the signal memory already exists in your neural network, ready to be triggered.

This is also why anesthesia works. Pain is processed by and can also be generated in the brain. If the pain of surgery did not need to be first sensed and processed by your brain, it wouldn't matter what drug you were given. Nothing would block the pain.

This also applies to the pain felt during traumatic events like a car accident, physical pain that surfaces during psychological therapy, and sometimes, depending on the origin, pain felt from conditions like migraines, stomach aches, and chronic pain. Depending on the reason for the pain, oftentimes there's no distinction between mental and physical, medical or psychological. The mind that observes isn't remotely choosing what to observe at all. It's ability for attention is modulated by, yep, you guessed it, the salience network.

The mind/body connection is also at the root of ailments that do not have identifiable medical causes. The search for the cause of a patient's symptoms typically involves multiple doctor's office visits, expensive tests, insurance claims, and in extreme cases, exploratory surgeries (sometimes at the patient's insistence) as the doctors search for a physical problem. After enough poking, prodding, slicing open, rooting around, and sewing back up again, still with no definitive answers, these individuals are sometimes accused of "imagining" their symptoms.

But they're not making it up. The problem is not in the body, detached from the brain. The problem is in the brain and the signals the brain is generating. The patient may really be feeling all the sensations and symptoms they're reporting, and a lot of the time those signals coming from the brain have psychological and emotional triggers.

When people are depressed, they feel more physical pain. When people are stressed out, they feel more physical pain. One stressful thought such as, "My girlfriend's about to break up with me," "My child just got an F on her test," "I'm afraid I might lose my job," or "I may have said the wrong thing in that conversation," can set off the stress switch. And boom! Physical pain can get fired up with the thought immediately. It's a very predictable pattern.

The gut is where most people feel the impact of stress, and Irritable Bowel Syndrome (IBS) is often stress-related. My pediatric patients with IBS have been scoped, tested, poked and prodded, given elimination diets, drugs, supplements, and just about every other remedy to try to fix their chronic stomach pain and gastrointestinal distress. Guess what happens once we lower their anxiety? The IBS goes away. There is a very long list of medical conditions that, in the absence of stress, remit completely or stop activating.

There's a vague recommendation many medical doctors give their patients. It goes something like this: "Make sure you manage your stress." This is excellent advice so far as it acknowledges stress as a powerful moderator of most illness. However, what does that mean? Usually people go back to trying to control their habitual sympathetic nervous responses with conscious thinking, and they ultimately fail at trying to outwit stress. Hopefully by reading this you're starting to see that managing stress the old-fashioned way is going to fall short. But don't worry—I've got your back.

Controlling the Uncontrollable

How does your nervous system actually function in relation to this connection between your mind and body? How much control do you really have?

Try this exercise. Notice your breathing right now, and notice you've been breathing this whole time you've been reading (and actually your whole life). I know this because you're still alive, right? You've been breathing without thinking about it. If you had to think about it consciously, you wouldn't have the mental capacity to do anything else. Inhaling and exhaling would be your entire life.

Fortunately, your autonomic (involuntary) nervous system regulates processes like breathing, which frees you up to make decisions, plan, work, fall in love, travel, and enjoy life. It's that powerful. But just to make the point that your autonomic nervous system is involuntary and operates beyond your control, let's try and override it anyway.

First, notice your breathing. Go ahead and take a deep breath. Assuming your stress switch isn't firmly in the on position, you'll be able to do that. (If it is, you will not. And if it is, it's probably a lot harder to comprehend these words right now). Now, stop breathing and don't start again until I tell you.

I have conducted this experiment in front of tens of thousands of people over the years in presentations. I announce to the audience, "I will give you a million dollars if you do not breathe until I tell you to start breathing again." About thirty seconds after this, a wave of chuckling will spread through the audience as everyone realizes how impossible that is to do.

Then, every once in a while, I'll get a former Olympic swimmer and they'll still be standing there with a smirk, long after the rest have gasped for air, chest puffed out proudly, still holding their breath. That's great, Mr. Elite Athlete, but before you go out and treat yourself to a flatbed truck of shiny new Speedos with my million-dollar prize money, I have a newsflash for you. The reason you didn't drop dead right there on the stage is NOT because you've outsmarted your autonomic nervous system completely. It's because you've trained your lungs over years of practice to have a longer capacity. Even an Olympic swimmer's autonomic nervous system will eventually kick in, once he reaches his own capacity for holding his breath.

Conscious training can get you so far, but ONLY so far, whereas a tool that works on the autonomic level could short-circuit the entire response. You can do your conscious best to control your breathing, and even stop your breathing momentarily. You have a conscious override. But that override is temporary, and it's not nearly as powerful as your autonomic system, which will eventually default to, "Sorry, my job is to make sure that you, as an organism, survive. I am turning the breathing switch back on and, by the way, you don't even know I'm doing it."

Presumably while you were reading all of this, you began breathing again and you're still with me. Now, can you tell me the exact moment when you started breathing again? Most likely, a you didn't even notice! Your brain made your body start breathing without your intent or your awareness. When I do this exercise, people don't usually consciously know when they started breathing again. If I ask someone when they think they did, they are oftentimes proven wrong when we check video. When we try to observe when our autonomic processes turn on again after we consciously tried to turn them off, we are usually wrong, because the autonomic system is involuntary, and therefore is not reliant on our consciousness. It operates outside of it. When you attempt to control your autonomic nervous system, you're trying to use conscious thought to control something that, by design, operates without your conscious control. This is the why the lizard brain wins over the executive brain over and over again.

When your stress switch is on, trying to exert conscious control over anything is usually an ineffective strategy unless you've practiced it over and over again; even then, the best strategies can break down.

A few years ago, I was at the Wisdom 2.0 Conference in San Francisco talking to a psychologist/meditation expert about what it would really take to override the stress response. Naturally the subject of meditation came up.

Tongue-in-cheek, I said, "Meditation is great over time and with lots of practice, but who has seven years to meditate in Tibet?"

With a serious look he responded, "I spent seven years of my life meditating in Tibet."

At that moment, I swore I heard Homer Simpson saying, "DOH!" inside my head, but luckily I had the inhibitory control to appear outwardly focused (and thus moderately intelligent).

I believed him, because this man had an incredible presence and was remarkably centered in the moment. He was the real deal. He was calm, thoughtful, and focused. Certainly the years of meditation had paid off for him.

Yes, experienced meditators can use their conscious brain to gain more control over their autonomic nervous system, just as an Olympic athlete has gained more short-term control over his breath. But most of us do not or cannot make room for that level of mind/body practice in our lives. We just don't have seven years to meditate in Tibet. We need other strategies.

Breathing is inherently an autonomic function, but using techniques like meditation, I can consciously control it and breathe deeply for a short period of time. But I can only do that when I'm relatively calm, and I can't control it forever. My involuntary systems are more powerful than my conscious mind. They're designed to take over because my survival as a biological mechanism is the top priority. Survival is in my DNA and was programmed long before the evolution of our conscious thought. We've been evolving for millions of years, and conscious thinking only came on the scene a relatively short time ago in the context of our evolution as a species. Therefore, biologically speaking, consciousness is not as powerful as we think it is.

Beyond biology and neurology, involuntary survival responses also occur on the mind/body level. Speaking to the capabilities of the conscious mind, we're *not* our thoughts—because we can think about our thoughts. We now have plenty of evidence that there is an inherent connection between our physical and mental states. In each of us is our observer, who can only operate when we're calm and unstressed enough to observe ourselves.

Whenever you're in this observer state, you're flexing your observer muscles and practicing being an observer. If you practice doing this regularly enough, the resulting calm "state" in your brain becomes more of a permanent "trait." Over time, this practice essentially resets your brain's stress switch default. This is one of the biggest benefits of meditation that you have probably heard about—getting stressed less easily and less often.

It's true that regular meditation can create more of a calm default so you can create a more peaceful, less stressed out brain. To achieve this neurological shift in your brain, however, requires a lot of time, thoughtfulness, and an absolutely committed habitual practice. It is unlikely to happen in the casual, "when I remember to do it," "New Year's resolution" fashion.

Some people don't like meditating at all: it's often downright scary to observe the internal thoughts your mind gets up to when you aren't preoccupied. Some of those thoughts are pretty terrible. They're saying negative things, trying to get you to worry, and telling you that you're a bad person. Psychologists term these thoughts "ANTs," for "automatic negative thoughts," and just like ants, they can run amok and cause chaos. We all have a self-talk mechanism that we don't have control over—until we do. In the meantime, it can be very negative.

Basically, in neurological terms, when you quiet everything down and try to meditate, your salience network pays attention to your thoughts instead of the TV or whatever else is usually going on around you. What's in your thoughts can be pretty unpleasant or scary, and when things are unpleasant, your fear and memory networks can signal your stress switch on as negative thoughts start flooding through the gates, and you might even believe those thoughts: "Oh wow! Look at what's in here!" "I hate myself! I'm no good, I should have done this and shouldn't have done that, what if he's upset with me, what if..." The barrage of unchecked thoughts can be really distressing.

And if you haven't practiced separating yourself from those thoughts so that you can observe and consider them, then simply becoming aware of them can activate the stress switch into full-blown fight-or-flight mode. The distress created by noticing negative thoughts can even become embedded into your fear system and your memory system. As a result, you may begin moving unconsciously away from your quiet, settled, focused, observer state. Because those negative thoughts become triggers for fear, triggers that your salience network will not block out, your unconscious mind will become even more motivated to keep you distracted. It wants you to stay so busy that avoidance patterns can develop.

There is a window here—a space between all of your thoughts and the ones you choose to believe—but you can't experience that space if your stress switch is on. Despite the potential for encountering negative thoughts, regular meditation or similar mind/body connective practices like deep breathing can be helpful: over time, they can reset the stress switch's default setting in the brain. They can create an awareness of the separation between those negative thoughts and how you choose to respond to them. Eventually, you can even prevent those thoughts from being automatically generated in the first place, so you won't need to use time and energy trying to manage them. But don't worry if you don't want to meditate—I am going to give you other options for how to short-circuit the problems described here.

All those medical issues that we've proven can be triggered by stress—from phantom limb pain to physical sensations and symptoms like migraines and irritable bowel syndrome—are proof positive that, sorry, Mr. Descartes, the mind and body do not live on separate islands that float independently in the middle of the ocean. They operate in one interconnected network and the idea they are split has served to confuse everyone about how the stress switch works.

Triggered

Within the interconnected mind/body network, the stress we experience in our bodies is triggered by a change in stimulus from inside of us (thoughts or pain) or outside (sounds, smells, touch, etc.) These stimuli are sensed and integrated by the salience network, which decides to turn the stress switch on or off. A quick note: because these functions are separate but connected, and also because you're probably used to hearing the mind and body described as two independent entities, you will frequently see me referring to only one or the other, even though they are always integrated and influenced by each other. Our bodies are internally connected and connected with things around us too.

In the mind/body, stress and its triggers are subjective to the individual. There are things that will set off anyone's stress switch, like seeing a snake about to strike, and there are also triggers that are unique to each person's stress system. Yet many people make an assumption that if certain things happen in their lives they should be stressed out; and conversely, they have a mental list of things that they believe shouldn't be stressful.

One college student could earn a C grade and be ecstatic about it, and another one could be extremely upset for days. Therefore, the idea that the same external trigger or event has the same effect on two different individuals' nervous systems is simply not true. The assumption that certain things should *not* cause stress is also false. An event or situation that would not cause stress for one person might well be a trigger for someone else.

This is why there is no place for the word "should" when assessing stress. If there's an external event that triggers the stress switch, we deal with what is—their stress switch is ON. We accept that something has caused stress, and in doing so we give the individual and others around them permission to do the same. There is no therapeutic value in trying to rationalize, deflect, or deny the presence of stress. The only appropriate response is to deal with it. Stress is not a hallucination, an excuse, or a personal weakness. And each individual's triggers are unique.

Any time we're in love relationships, we're particularly vulnerable to situations relating to the relationship that can trigger our stress response. I've had some very distressed women come in for counseling because their husbands had emotional affairs. In one case, the husband was talking to a colleague at work, sharing things about his life, and even turning to this other woman for emotional support. In doing so, he built a communication barrier between himself and his wife. Sometimes this kind of relationship turns physical, but even when it doesn't, for many women, this can trigger incredible stress and in some cases even cause PTSD. Then, rather than direct their anger at their husbands, these women beat themselves about the fact that they're allowing themselves to be stressed, rationalizing, "Why should I be upset about this? He didn't get physical with her!"

The truth of the matter is that this is a very common trigger of nervous system reactivity that needs to be addressed—and even if it was unique to one person, it would need to be addressed. If the stress is ignored and the situation not processed, things can totally break down between the couple. And without resolution, this woman's nervous system could continue to be triggered daily, leaving her wondering if she is crazy. No amount of "should" will provide her with relief. The stress switch needs to be dealt with.

The cure for stress and the reactivity it has triggered does not reside not in a person's consciousness. This surprises so many people who think they can outwit stress. With the right facts, the well-meaning person reasons, the trigger can be banished, a stressed out person can find relief, and normal life can resume. Although they mean well, this is simply unrealistic. The nervous system just doesn't work that way.

Try telling someone with an elevator phobia: "Hey! This elevator is safe. No one's ever gotten stuck in this elevator. And we're only going to go one floor up."

The phobic person is standing there frozen in front of the elevator, deciding whether or not to get in it, while their nervous system is sending very clear signals that if they step foot in that elevator, they're going to die. They are in full fight-or-flight, sweating, heart pounding, out of breath, pupils dilated. Their phobia of elevators has completely triggered their nervous system, and this chain reaction is now well beyond their control.

Using logic and reason and other tactics that require higher-order mental functioning is pretty useless in that moment. Standing there in front of that elevator, you might as well be trying to have a calm, rational conversation with a lizard brain attached to a live electric wire. Save your breath.

Even if you were to physically force the phobic person into the elevator (which wouldn't be a particularly kind thing to do, by the way) their level of reactivity would only ratchet up higher, since now you've moved the live wire even closer to the electric source. All you would accomplish would be to strengthen the trigger and reinforce their phobic pattern.

There are some therapies that incorporate graduated exposure to lower the anxiety response, but these are time-intensive and require a commitment to face the fear, which many people won't do because—you guessed it—the stress switch is in control.

Once the fear system is locked onto a trigger (the sight of an elevator), unless we desensitize the stress switch in that situation, it's going to stay. This is why anxiety, phobias, and other fears usually get worse without treatment. First the fear system locks onto one trigger, and then it expands to more and more triggers over time. That's when the individual starts avoiding the trigger and everything related to it as a survival strategy. A phobia of elevators can progress to a fear of entering tall buildings, then to all buildings, then in extreme cases, to going out in public at all. The individual narrows down their world down to try to stay safe based on their nervous system's shrinking assessment of what's safe and what's not in the world. Their salience network signals fear too often, activating the stress switch and essentially telling them that they have to avoid, avoid, avoid. There's often no way for someone to consciously think themselves out of this vicious cycle without help.

In these situations, most people can't turn off the stress switch with conscious thoughts. A person with anxiety can certainly try to rationalize, "There's nothing to be afraid of. I'm just going to do it. I'm going to get into that elevator (or on that plane, or out of the house, or to the grocery store, etc.)." But as soon as they attempt it, the stress switch turns on, and their rational, executive brain is powerless to the force of millions of years of biological evolution. This person is not weak; they are simply human, and their body is doing what it was designed to do—survive. In the face of that biological imperative, our executive brain, our thinking mind, what we might even call consciousness, is fighting an uphill battle, and usually losing.

Nevertheless, we're obsessed with consciousness. Obsessed with it! We love the idea that we have all this behavioral control, and that our consciousness is so powerful that we can do all these great things just by harnessing our mind's power. We believe that we've evolved way past our mechanical involuntary bodies and lizard brains.

I'm sorry to have to tell you this, but most of your behavior, reactions, and body sensations are controlled by pre-conscious brain networks operating without your awareness. Remember, that's good news, because if we needed consciousness for those hundreds and thousands of body functions, we wouldn't have the mind power to build skyscrapers, create art, solve problems, invent things, cure diseases, and all those other beautiful, high-level activities. We would be just regulating ourselves the whole time without any mind power to spare. Fortunately, evolution has found a balance between pre-conscious and conscious processes that allows us to function well in our daily lives.

The fallout happens when we confuse the roles of biology and consciousness, including in our approach to treating stress. We've all had that experience of thinking, "Ugh! I know I shouldn't be upset about this thing. Logically, I know I shouldn't be upset but every time I think about I, get all riled up!"

The problem is, you're trying to apply conscious logic to a nervous system reaction. No matter how rational and logical you consider yourself to be, certain situations will cause that stress switch to be set off.

I've had well-meaning parents come in with their heads hanging down, with mom saying, "I love my son, I do, but I can't stop yelling at him because he does these things that just drive me up the wall. I know logically it's not a big deal, yet every time he does it, I just lose it! What is wrong with me?"

I tell her, "There's nothing wrong with you. There's a mismatch between the power of your stress switch and your conscious ability to control it. All this means is that you are human, and what we need to do is make these things not trigger the switch. We'll do that by processing certain things in the memory networks so you don't have to keep dealing with getting set off. Then we can decide how you want to handle your son's behavior."

Why do we need to dig into the memory networks? (And I'm not talking about poking or prodding anything—we can do this with EMDR therapy). Well, your fear and memory systems dictate more behavior than you'd like to think they do, and it's important that they buddy up to help with your survival.

Let's say that as a child you went for a walk in the woods, accidentally stumbled over a beehive, tumbled onto the ground, and a swarm of bees descended on you, leaving you with dozens of painful welts all over your body. Now, because of the emotional charge attached to that memory, your fear system is locked into the experience. Your fear and memory systems will work together, sending you unconscious signals to keep you out of that situation in the future. Their job is to manage your automatic survival programming and keep you from getting attacked by a swarm of bees again. The signals may cause choices that seem irrational, creating, for example, a nervous system trigger that makes you afraid of going for any walks in the woods. This system may go really far, even signaling the need to avoid all outdoor situations, or create an outright phobia of the outdoors. But again, these systems aren't designed to make sense to your conscious mind. Their sole job is your survival.

Together they work to power the stress switch on in situations where there might be bees, so you don't go around falling into beehives over and over again. This learning mechanism can work great to avoid dangers to your survival, but if they are overactive, they can make you fearful when you don't really need to be. Your fear and memory systems, as illogical as they seem sometimes, are looking out for you.

On a lesser scale, can you think of certain things in your life that you want to do but for some reason you avoid? Maybe you've always wanted to go camping, surfing, traveling overseas, dancing. If fear or avoidance overrides what could be an otherwise fun and pleasant experience, it's likely that at some point, your fear and memory systems teamed up in response to something that happened in your life, and an unconscious avoidance mechanism was formed. You might not even have noticed until just now when I brought it to your attention, because it's embedded in your autonomic nervous system, dictating your behavior while making you believe your avoidance behaviors are perfectly logical. That's the joint power of the fear and memory systems: when they work together, they keep you alive, but sometimes they go too far.

Ditch the Guilt

Now that you understand that your conscious thoughts are really no match for your salience network's ability to turn on your stress switch without your awareness, you can ditch any negative thoughts you have about yourself for being unable to control your stress.

You can breathe more easily, because you understand there are neurological reasons why you can't just outwit stress the way you've been trying to (with the possible exception of those of you who have seven years to spend meditating in Tibet). There are real, scientific reasons why you can't outwit your stress, and neither can your co-workers, your boss, your friends, your family, your husband, or your children. So we can stop blaming each other and ourselves.

This is worth repeating: you are not flawed for not being able to control stress as you've been trying to do. You are human. So let's honor the neurological basis of your humanity and move forward.

Now that you know this, let's talk about how the medical system views your stress and what they think you should do about it. And don't worry, afterwards I will teach you how to short-circuit your stress switch and live into your best life.

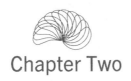

Chapter Two

DUPED!

I have my own story to tell about pain and the mind/body connection. In my thirties I had unexplained back pain that persisted for eight years. Since there was no obvious cause, I believed for a long time that it would go away, but eventually I sought medical advice. As a doctor, I initially put my trust in the system that I've long been a part of, naturally expecting a solution for my temporary condition. In my mind, the back pain I had been experiencing for eight years should have been a solvable problem. In the minds of my doctors, it was not.

I was shocked when, after seeing a number of doctors, surgeons, and specialists, I was informed that my back pain was caused by a "chronic condition." Medical professionals agreed that mine was not a problem that could be solved, and I should learn to live with it, like millions of other Americans saddled with the diagnosis of "chronic illness." To me, this felt like the medical system throwing up their collective hands and saying, "We've got nothing for you. Chin up, carry on and live the best you can with this monkey on your back."

They proposed surgery followed by a lifetime of pills to control the pain—to merely cope. Doctors handed down a sentence of chronic back pain and a mandate to stop one of my greatest joys in life, running. Worst of all, they acknowledged helplessly that this incurable pain-restricted life would also affect my ability to be the best mom I could be to my two small children.

I was upset and frustrated. I'm a doctor devoted to curing people of stress and moving beyond false limitations. Being told, "we can't fix this—you just have to live with it," was not okay with me. While the medical establishment all parroted the same dreadful outcome for me, I refused to own this new "chronic pain patient" label and all its implications for my life and freedom. Chronic pain is an invisible leash that allows you to move through life, but always with the knowledge that if you forget the leash is there and run too freely, you will be yanked back. It keeps you from living at your full potential.

Before committing to invasive surgery and a lifetime of chemical dependency, I looked hard for someone who might disagree. I saw a number of physical therapists for pain relief, hoping someone could offer a different solution. And I finally found one! When I described my chronic pain to this new therapist, he believed we could eliminate it. In his words, it would be "easy-peasy" to fix my pain, permanently. Easy-peasy? How had the very same back condition gone from completely unsolvable to easy-peasy?

My new easy-peasy PT and personal superhero educated me about what was going on with my back, and recommended a combination of alternative treatments including dry needling, yin yoga, and specific exercises every day for a few weeks, required I take some long-term action on my part in a way that fit my lifestyle, such as stretching and massages, and I was on my way. These treatments—that the established medical community did not offer—worked for me. I can run twelve to fifteen miles a week again, and I have a minimal amount of pain. No surgery, no chemical dependency.

At first I was ecstatic and relieved, and ready to get back to my morning runs. Life was good again. But then I started reviewing the long road I'd traveled from the diagnosis of incurable chronic pain to, finally, an easy-peasy cure. I moved from frustrated to completely stupefied that I had been told nothing could be done. How could medical providers sell me a bill of goods, saddling me with a chronic, incurable diagnosis for a condition that actually was treatable?

I thought about what might have happened if I had accepted their permanent diagnosis, embedded the "chronic pain" label into my identity, quit the physical activities I love most, and held my best self back from my children. My blood boiled. How dare they? How dare they try to take my life away with status quo messages? And I also seethed at the possibility that alternative solutions might have been concealed in the name of profit, since patients with chronic conditions can easily become veritable cash cows for the system.

But then I calmed down and came to my senses. As a reasonable human being and a doctor with a PhD in neuropsychology, I believe it is irrational to conclude that the well-meaning physicians who told me they couldn't fix my back pain intentionally avoided offering non-surgical solutions. Contrary to some popular opinions, those doctors themselves were not out to get me or my wallet. I really believe that my physicians were convinced they were acting in my best interests, according to the collective oath to do no harm, and that they treated me the only way they knew how, based on the western medical system. The doctors who diagnosed my pain as chronic did so because that's the paradigm they're working from. Unfortunately, as players in a system that treats chronic conditions the exact wrong way, they've been duped.

But the near-sightedness of the medical establishment isn't stopping millions of Americans from investing their trust and hard earned dollars into this broken system. Who can blame them? We've all been conditioned from a young age that when you're sick you go to the doctor, and the doctor makes you better. And back pain is just one example of the many chronic conditions that conventional medicine is complacent about. Believe it or not the most frequently treated, most expensive, most prevalent and most destructive chronic condition overwhelming the medical system and the world is stress. And within our conventional medical system, the most predominant way to make anxiety better is in the form of a pill.

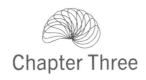

Chapter Three

HOOKED!

In order to get a feel for the size of the problem, consider the following stunning statistics about pharmaceutical-based treatments for stress:

A 2013 study found that one in six U.S. adults reported taking a psychiatric drug such as an antidepressant or a sedative.[6]

In 2010, Americans spent more than $16 billion on antipsychotics, $11 billion on antidepressants and $7 billion for drugs to treat attention deficit hyperactivity disorder (ADHD).[7]

The Stress Disconnect

To understand why medications are the system's first line answer to anxiety, we first need to understand the paradigm they're working from. Let me be Captain Obvious for a moment and say that doctors do actually understand quite a bit about how the human brain and body works. As students, we study the outer and inner workings for years, down to the molecular level, sleepless school night after sleepless school night. The systemic disconnect around stress is not because doctors don't get it—believe me, we get it. The issue is in the language western medicine uses to categorize stress. Somewhere between our knowledge of how the brain works, our interpretation of what stress is, and our translations to the public, the language of stress has been incorrectly twisted into noise and confusion that makes treating it very difficult.

Stress is a short-term state inside of the body triggered by sensory input from outside the body or internal signals. The stress switch is triggered by stressors like loud sounds, seeing a snake, having an "oh no!" thought, or touching a sharp object. Chronic stress is basically a stress switch that is too sensitive and turns on over and over again. If left untreated, this turning on can become almost continuous, playing out like the same scene of a movie, over and over. When this happens, rather than being a short-term problem with a clear solution, it becomes a long-term disorder playing out day after day.

As a systemic issue, the problem is not that this long-term disorder isn't fixable; the problem is that we accept that we have to live with it as a part of reality. You wouldn't decide the busted water pipe in your basement is impossible to fix, get a raft, and adapt to life in your new watery reality. So why do we think we have to live with chronic stress?

In the medical world, this often looks like a patient going to the doctor, already deep into the replay loop, with stress poisoning all corners of her life, like that toxic mercury in the pond. In this scenario, the doctor looks at the complexity of his patient's condition and translates this stress, not as a solvable problem with an immediate solution, but rather as an entire disorder that, because of its complexity, she'll likely suffer from for life. Now, this patient has a disease, and the medical system shuffles people with a disease into the disease model of care. There's the treatment area, populated with nice, straightforward, fixable cases of broken bones and respiratory infections. Then there's the disease area, filled with the incurables, whose best hope is temporary symptom relief.

For this patient, her disease diagnosis is chronic stress, so now she's in a group with the other chronically ill people (chronic pain, asthma, migraines, autoimmune disorders, etc.). Her doctor—and in all probability any other doctors she sees—will treat her according to the thinking that this is a lifelong condition, a cure is not possible, and therefore, the goal is relief from symptoms.

The doctor feels satisfied, having diagnosed the problem, sorted the patient into the disease paradigm he knows and trusts, and created the very best care plan for his patient that his knowledge (and her insurance) can buy.

The patient will learn to adapt to this new label of "chronic stress patient." What other choice does she have? Some variations of this label include generalized anxiety disorder, post-traumatic stress disorder, obsessive-compulsive disorder, social anxiety disorder, and phobic disorder. Each patient takes ownership of their disorder with the specificity of the label they have been assigned. The label will also appease the insurance companies, generating a code that signifies there's a real problem, and in this case, a problem deemed chronic or permanent that requires ongoing treatments designed to manage it.

Meanwhile, after the sorting and labeling is complete, this particular patient will embark on a new and never-ending journey of medicating and managing her stress as this monkey on her back, because this is how her condition has been translated to her in the language of disease. This will be her new reality, and she'll learn to live with it. This is how a broken water pipe that can be easily repaired becomes a person floating around on a raft in a flooded house, adapting to their new reality. Because they've been duped into believing it.

Do No Harm

The system plays a significant role in propagating this lie. It is an enabler of sorts, reinforcing the message that since stress is not curable, it's your job to accept it and make it manageable. It's your monkey; learn to tame it.

The reality is that people are diagnosed with many lifelong chronic problems that are neither lifelong nor chronic at all. For stress in particular, the right combination of treatments can send the monkey packing.

As I mentioned earlier, most doctors are ethical, good-hearted, well-intentioned professionals who are certainly not trying to fool people into staying sick. In and of themselves, many different medical treatments for stress can be effective. I am not against any of them, including what for some people is public enemy #1—prescription drugs. Prescription medications have been historically successful in treating and managing many different chronic diseases, including anxiety. The problem comes when the prescription pad becomes the go-to solution even when it really isn't a great solution at all. When all you have is a hammer, everything looks like a nail.

Many people today are acquiring prescriptions for medications from their doctors without being aware that counseling, therapy, and other treatments such as those mentioned in this book often have higher rates of success. One study found that many people are being prescribed medications from their primary care doctors without being aware that other treatments such as therapy have higher rates of success.[8] A pill may be an easy and time-efficient answer, but it is not always the safest or most effective way to help someone.

I want to reiterate: this doesn't mean that the prescribing physicians are intending to do harm. It means that they have been trained within a medical system that is slanted toward chemical solutions for medical problems. And as anyone who has ever taken medication for an extended period of time with no real success can tell you, even when medications seem like the hammer, we've often misidentified the nail.

Chuck

Chuck was taking a benzodiazepine for sleep and Prozac for anxiety. I learned that a doctor had put him on both drugs FIVE years earlier, when Chuck was having a hard time coping with his father's death. Now he was coming to me for relief from the side effects. He was unmotivated, forty pounds overweight, and had very little sex drive. I asked him if he'd had any history of anxiety, depression, or sleep problems prior to his father's death. None. His doctor's treatment for a short-term problem had become a long-term solution, and now that he was hooked on the pills and saddled with the side effects, I had a whole new, and much more insidious, problem to solve for this patient. I had to get him off the medications so he could get his life back.

This is easier said than done. If you have even a basic understanding of pharmaceutical withdrawal, you probably know that getting off of medications, especially after a long period of time, can be very difficult. This patient was facing the reality of a short-term rebound so unpleasant that many people find the experience intolerable. Many can't handle it and ultimately decide to stay on the medications unless we can ease the transition.

Medication withdrawal can be like the movie *Castaway* where Tom Hanks' character has to get over an enormous wave in order to break free from the island. Living on a deserted island is a terrible long-term fate, but as one violent wave after another smacks him down while he tries to break through to calmer waters, it seems it would be very easy to give up. That's what it's like to come off of many medications aimed to relieve stress: trying to escape but getting smacked in the face by giant waves over and over. It was my job to get this patient off medication island.

Was it the doctor's intention to get Chuck hooked on medications for the long-term, eventually having to face painful withdrawal? Absolutely not. If I had gone back and asked that doctor what he was thinking, he probably would have told me, "Look, this person came to me in grave distress—he wasn't sleeping, wasn't eating, and his work and relationships were suffering. He had no quality of life. I prescribed him a medication and recommended he go to therapy, do yoga, and a few other ways to get relief beyond the medication I prescribed. That's all I had time to do in the fifteen minutes I had with him. And when he came back for a med check a few months later, I had even less time. All I could ask was how the prescriptions were helping, he said fine, he was feeling better and sleeping better. That was the best I could do for this patient in the time I had with him. I told him other things to do like yoga and therapy, but he never followed through on those."

So do you see how even the most skilled, well-intentioned physician is hamstrung in a system where time is scarce, big dollars are on the line, and the goal is to get patients from complaint to treatment as quickly and efficiently as possible? This kind of system philosophy is the exact opposite of what works for chronic anxiety patients, as well as patients with any other chronic, long-term condition. Short-term, simple fixes (that often aren't even great fixes) are complete fails for long-term, complicated problems. To be told otherwise, to be given the impression that the solution you are receiving is the *only* solution to your problem, and that you must accept it, is to be duped.

The good news is that we were able to get Chuck off of medication island by combining neurofeedback, EMDR therapy, TouchPoints, and other methods. He's now better than ever! He's lost almost all of the excess weight he gained on the medication and is happy and healthy. Using these techniques, he was able to process the grief of losing his father that, even on the medication, was still affecting him daily, and is doing very well.

Zealots

Extremes rarely work, especially as a remedy for complex problems like chronic disorders. Just like the psychiatrists who prescribed medications to ninety-nine percent of their patients, completely rejecting all medications across the board is also not the solution.

But don't tell that to the many Americans who have completely rejected traditional medicine, catapulted themselves outside the thick steel walls of the system, and have made it their life's mission to immerse themselves in alternative solutions. It's incredible how much people invest in extreme stress relief programs that have questionable results because they are too defiant to accept the most effective solutions.

In my neuropsychology practice I've seen parents spend up to thirty thousand dollars on a bevy of remedies that failed, but justify the time and money wasted as okay because "at least it's all natural." In their minds, I believe they think they're progressive and forward thinking, and these extreme investments they're making are to outsiders and alternative medicine providers whom they characterize as the good guys, out to "stick it to the man." You've seen that I'm as frustrated with the system as anyone else, and possibly more so because of my position as a part of it. But the solution to this frustration is *not* some fanatical, across-the-board, blatant rejection of all modern western medicine including all pharmaceuticals.

Rather than seeking out the good and effective remedies available in both conventional and alternative medicine, zealots are swayed by misinformation, fascinated with the unproven, romanticized by personal success stories from alternative remedies, and of course, motivated to find a cure for themselves or their child. I will never fault this motivation, but I will always question the choices that stem from it.

It's well known that the top treatments for ADHD are medication and neurofeedback. When I dare mention medication to some parents, I am quickly cut down with rhetoric, such as "I don't want to teach my child that pills are the answer!" And agreed, I don't want to teach people that pills are the *only* answer, nor do I think they should be prescribed when other solutions could work. However, medication can be a part of a comprehensive plan, and without medications, sometimes we can't reach certain goals.

I explain to these well-meaning parents, "I don't want your children to grow up failing school, being an outcast, repeating a grade, generally not thriving and developing a sense of identity that they're a terrible person, and later getting on (illegal) drugs." Studies find that teens with ADHD who do not take medication for it cause four times more car accidents than teens without ADHD or teens with ADHD that is treated with medication. This is how an extremist approach against medical treatment can risk lives. These parents will try discipline, threats, essential oils, and supplements, all without good outcomes, but will reject completely some things that have been shown to work. I agree that when there's a non-pharmaceutical solution that's can be as effective as medication, let's do that first. For example, for certain problems, neurofeedback can be an effective alternative—but in the cases that it doesn't work, let's not reject medication altogether—especially given the car accidents and other dangers to untreated children and teens.

Similarly to conventional medical doctors who intend to do no harm, I believe these parents are obviously not trying to harm their children by their mindset. Some of their rejection of western medicine in favor of total, unconditional embrace of any other alternative comes from utter information overwhelm. Overwhelming marketing dollars contribute to simply too much confusion and noise when it comes to treatment options. It's very, very hard to tease out the snake oil from the rest.

One product of—and contributor to—the information overwhelm about treatment options is a newer phenomenon called biohacking. One expert has described biohacking as, "a new and emerging movement of amateurs conducting life sciences outside of traditional professional settings such as university and corporate labs."[9]

Based on my firsthand observations, biohackers attempt to tweak their biology in various ways for desired effects, and then blog about what works so others can replicate their experiments and see if they get the same results. However, a key missing piece of the biohacking puzzle is the reality that every one of us has unique biology that reacts differently to various modes of treatment. This is why the FDA requires pharmaceutical companies to run clinical trials on large numbers of people: to make sure that possible benefits exceed the placebo effect and, not insignificantly, to examine any unwanted side effects. Pharmaceuticals are designed to be a ratio of one solution for many people. Biohacking experiments are a ratio of one solution to one person, and later, maybe it will work for other people, too. But who really knows what will happen until they try it?

On a one-to-one basis, we are all biohackers in a way—experimenting through the process of trying different things to see what works to create a desired outcome. Think of the trends now: no gluten, no dairy, veganism/vegetarianism, large doses of vitamins and supplements, cleanses and detoxes, not to mention noninvasive mind/body techniques like yoga, tapping, and neuro-linguistic programming. This list goes on and on. We basically try something and see if it works for us.

Self-purported biohackers just do it with more zeal, in a public forum, and in some cases they track measurements. They'll drink elixirs, inject their bodies, and do all things in the name of science—sometimes while throwing caution about potential side effects to the wind. The problem with biohacking is that in some cases, you can't isolate variables to attribute cause.

I recently met with a well-known biohacker in Los Angeles to discuss non-invasive methods for treating stress (including TouchPoints) that he could track rather than some of the crazier, more invasive things he was trying. Some of these guys are like modern-day Jackasses (as in the television show), but he was a very intelligent, respectable guy. He described his method to me: "I try out different things and then I blog about them. I'm starting a wellness community." He had been experimenting with several supplements alongside other wellness products and health strategies, while blogging about his experience to his community.

The morning of our meeting, however, he was a mess. His face was red and broken out, he had a splitting headache, and he was massively dehydrated. He drank four glasses of water during our meeting! It was obvious to me that he'd been out partying the night before, and based on his symptoms, not just with alcohol. First, we had a little talk about the contradiction of trying to improve and destroy your health at the same time. Then, I pointed out that trying so many products and strategies at once without allowing enough time for any one thing to work, or to examine carefully measured results, was not the most effective way to successfully hack your biology.

But I also realized while talking to him that people will listen to biohackers and their personal stories, often giving their subjective "data" more weight than objective, research-based science. That's the reality of the information overwhelm; it becomes much easier to cherry-pick through the internet piles and believe whatever feels and sounds good over what has been actually proven to work.

People love rituals, personal stories, and information that aligns with their personal beliefs, experiences, and biases. People also love enthusiasm, and for that reason, please never underestimate the power of your brain's favorite pleasure chemical, dopamine. You've probably heard of or even attended network marketing conventions and self-help events that feature bright flashing lights, fireworks, loud music, happy people reveling in their love for certain products and celebrating the money they've ostensibly made selling them. All those exciting, flashy elements work together to turn your body into a dopamine factory. It's not a coincidence that these events are so much like a football game—there's togetherness, camaraderie, lots of people celebrating, loving life, and all supporting their favorite team. The professional sports industry is also a fan of dopamine. If someone could bottle up all the dopamine being released at any of those events and crop-spray it across America, we would be the happiest bunch of people on the planet. That sense of elation that comes with getting caught up in a trend is partially because of dopamine, and it can hijack all of our sensibilities when it comes to rational decision-making.

This creates a kind of group bias that can accumulate large numbers of believers. This phenomenon can make you try crazy things, and it also helps fuel an across-the-board rejection of all things conventional medicine for some people. Surround yourself with a trusted group of social media friends who seem to know what they're talking about, toss some seemingly legitimate wellness articles into the mix, sprinkle in some demonization of western medicine, place the entire scenario into the shadows of a feel-good, authoritative-sounding marketing campaign, and suddenly everything makes perfect sense.

Faulty conclusions can't help but follow all of that propaganda and dopamine. It all seems to make sense to us because of how our brains use heuristics (shortcuts) to make decisions. With all these pretty people, friend endorsements, biohackers, and salespeople touting an awesome new solution for what ails you, *of course* the right combination of essential oils can cure sciatica, lingering digestive disorder, and high blood pressure! And *of course* you don't need to worry about checking with a doctor when you combine a custom made cocktail of assorted supplements—after all, they are all *natural*, so they must be fine! That logic ignores the fact that lead and arsenic are one hundred percent natural too, and those are lethal. And if you read sarcasm here, you are on the right track. In my opinion, some of these remedies simply require a complete lack of common sense, or judgment, or both. I once went to a natural health store looking for supplements and a clerk recommended that I drink my own urine—and showed me multiple books as evidence!

Let's consider essential oils and supplements as examples, because these are two of the types of supposedly natural treatments that people are most hopped up about now. Few of the supplements and none of the oils are FDA-approved to treat any condition. Most users aren't entirely sure what's in any of them, whether they're dosing appropriately, or how they mix with each other. But people will eagerly take on these risks while insisting, "I refuse to take even one toxic pharmaceutical! But my friend said...." Or, "I heard that this natural supplement works great, so I'm going to try it..."

I have a brilliant friend who extols the virtues of taking magnesium and calcium supplements above all else. "I've done the research," she said, and directed me to a certain celebrity-backed wellness website. Because someone famous was behind it, and she trusted the source who sent her there, she was convinced. Sorry, but that's not research. We are biased to trust celebrities or athletes, and thus fail to confirm information in other ways. She was actually surprised the marketing content on the website didn't sway me to buy the supplements for myself! I often give presentations at professional conferences where rooms full of doctors will ask me what I recommend to patients for X or Y or Z; they will furiously write down this prescription, desperate for a sort of recipe that they will then use without all the knowledge or limits of how I apply it.

There's some research suggesting that people who freestyle with supplements in large doses have worse outcomes for their initial medical condition than those treated by pharmaceuticals. People who take excessive numbers and dosages of vitamins actually have a higher risk of certain cancers than others who do not. A twenty-year literature review presented at a 2015 meeting of the American Association for Cancer Research found an "overall increased risk of cancer among vitamin users," particularly in those who exceed the recommended dosages.[10]

However, when news of such research hits the folks who are rigidly tied to the natural remedy movement, the group translation is something like, "That's big pharma trying to keep you sick by keeping you away from natural supplements!" The whole group nods authoritatively on social media—and shares the post as a representation of scandal rather than a potentially credible finding.

Identifying with one side of two seemingly opposing groups creates natural bias that I'd like to help you shed so it doesn't get in the way of your judgment when you are making decisions about your health. Unlike being a fan of the Patriots vs. the Eagles, being on the conventional vs. holistic medical team doesn't have to be an either-or choice.

If you self-identify too completely with one 'camp' or way of thinking—whether it's holistic, natural, alternative, traditional, medical, or otherwise—you will become less objective in choosing potential solutions for what ails you. This happens on a large scale in the medical and psychological professions, where psychologists may often demonize any pharmaceutical treatments, while medical doctors are quick to question the effectiveness of anything non-pharmaceutical. Furthermore, the general public often overlooks the reality that supplements, herbs, and other kinds of "natural" treatments can affect chemical changes in the same ways as prescription drugs. Affiliating with a camp may also limit your thinking in terms of what's available. When the question is limited to, "do I take a pharmaceutical pill or a supplement," the larger question about whether invading the body with anything is the answer—or only part of the answer, or something to consider later—is totally lost in the shuffle.

I'm not immune to bias and choosing camps myself. Several years ago I wrote an article about how medication, therapy, and executive functioning coaching were the best treatments for ADHD and that I did not believe neurofeedback was very helpful. I had done a less-than-thorough job of researching neurofeedback, but I had some patients who had undergone the treatment and didn't get great results.

I followed the American Psychological Association's recommendations in my article and felt quite smug when they put my article next to a local neurofeedback practitioner's article extolling the virtues of neurofeedback for ADHD. The next week I had a patient come in who swore neurofeedback worked, but told me they underwent a different kind of neurofeedback—19-channel vs. 2-channel—which apparently has a more robust training effect.

I finally did a thorough literature review and had to recant. Whoops! I couldn't deny that when done correctly, neurofeedback was probably effective for a wide range of conditions—one of which was ADHD. I'm not so rigid that I would throw up a wall of psychological defenses after realizing I was wrong.

Instead I used it as a lesson, and told my team I was wrong to assume something didn't work based on a few reports and without really doing the research myself. I also made the mistake of clumping all kinds of neurofeedback under one heading and rejecting it all. It's the same thing with any of the endless things we can call "therapy"—some types of therapy are incredibly helpful, and some are simply not.

As a result of this lesson, I'm now conscious that our science in general is evolving, and I'm evolving in my knowledge. What I tell you today may shift and change based on new information, evolving science, or improved technology, and we all have to put on our big-girl and big-boy pants and say "whoops" every once in a while. I don't care how many letters you have after your name.

The moral of my humbling professional story is to note how quickly, in the face of conflicting information, I was willing to go back, do a whole new literature review, and essentially take back my original conclusion. This level of rigorous evidence-based research, the willingness to admit when you are wrong, and the extra effort required to correct your mistake and publicly apologize, is what is missing in the rigid, zealous thinking that is so prevalent everywhere today. I am not questioning the motives of people who seek health solutions, whether they look inside or outside of the conventional system. I understand completely that every single person who is seeking any cure is simply trying to feel better and live a better life. Many have been burned by the same medical system that burned me. I get it.

But if you are firmly rooted in any one extreme of how to treat what ails you, I encourage you to develop a more discriminating point of view. Reject what doesn't work, always seek the truth, and pull back the curtain when you're being duped. Be willing to question anyone, whether it's the doctor telling you there's no cure or the wellness guru telling you to drink your own pee. After that, keep seeking solutions to your problem without ruling out anything based on social bias, subjective personal stories from others, or what you think you know. Cures are out there and extreme, zealot-like thinking only blocks potential paths to healing.

Hope

I still can't believe how close I came to accepting as fact the lie that I would be in debilitating pain for the rest of my life. I can't believe I let myself live with eight years of back pain, when as it turned out, there was such a simple solution. It took me awhile to find Mr. Easy–peasy the physical therapist. I endured dozens of treatments that didn't work along the way—dollar after dollar shelled out, hours and hours at appointment after appointment squeezed into my busy life, with mounting frustration that nothing was working. I lost hope at times, in my lowest moments thinking, "Maybe they're right. Maybe I just have to live with my back pain. I've tried everything and nothing is working." I was exhausted, living my life on a leash, and ready to give up. It took everything left within me to continue on, to fight, until I finally found a physical therapist who combined his treatments with a solid plan for what I needed to do, and it cured me.

I understand how people in my situation, diagnosed with a seemingly incurable condition, get to this place. You may honestly believe you've tried it all, because it really feels like you have.

But the reality is you *haven't* tried it all. If you're still suffering and not getting acceptable results, I want you to know that there may be a better way out there—a trustworthy professional who can give you real results or a method that really works. Your life, health, and happiness depend on believing that there are no dead ends. The system might have failed you so far, but there is good news. It's time for a change, a paradigm shift about "chronic" conditions, starting with the biggest one of all, the one at the heart of it all—stress.

You may be feeling frustrated and even hopeless, like I was, baffled by a system that's telling you the best you can hope for is to cope with your stress; that it's incurable, and you are powerless to change that.

In the meantime, even coping gets more and more difficult. The stress you're dealing with in your life, and the stress you watch others go through, is not letting up. Just when you think you've gotten a handle on it, something else happens, and you feel like you're right back where you started. Maybe it wakes you up in the middle of the night, gripping your brain with a torrent of thoughts that don't seem to have an off switch. Or perhaps it sends you into a panic of anxiety whenever you're around large groups of people. Maybe without warning, your stress switch sends you into emotionally jarring flashbacks from past traumatic situations, some even dating back to your childhood. The chain reaction can have you suffering—and could have your partner or your children suffering—and nobody has a solution for you. This idea that you are stuck with stress for the rest of your life might feel too overwhelming to handle sometimes.

I get it. That's why we're having this conversation right now. I'm here to present NEW solutions, and ones that won't drain your bank account and fill your calendar with endless treatments and obligations, all in the name of merely coping. Together, we can mobilize our frustrations with both the broken medical system and the extreme alternatives that also haven't solved the problem. It's time to take action. The paradigm shift begins here and now!

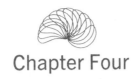

Chapter Four

COPING VS. CURING: A NEW PARADIGM

Doctors do not like to talk about a cure.
~Fredric Neuman, MD

Alicia, age twenty-two, was living her life held hostage on a battlefield of panic attacks. She came to me for help coping with the explosions of panic she tripped like landmines when venturing out in public places like the grocery store, movies, concerts—anywhere she might encounter other people. By time I met her, she was seriously considering giving up driving for fear of having another panic attack in the car. Like many patients, Alicia's medical doctor had told her she the panic attacks were a lifelong disorder, one that she could manage with a drug, Xanax. As a result, Alicia believed she had no other choice but to expect panic attacks in public, using medication to lessen their severity enough to at least continue functioning at a basic level. I thought that sounded like a pretty crummy prognosis, especially for a twenty-two year-old with her whole life in front of her.

I told Alicia, "Panic is like a landmine exploding. Containing it when it happens is really hard, and it's no wonder you want to avoid life situations where you fear stepping on a mine. But what if we could get rid of the tripwires that set off the explosions, so you can roam freely within your life, regardless of what you find?"

Now I agree that until we cured the panic, Alicia would need to find ways to cope, but I didn't want her story to end there.

When you're stressed, your lizard brain is in control, and it wants you to cope by avoiding situations where you may encounter landmines, which shrinks the scope of your life. If you try to negotiate with your irrational, lizard brain about walking into a field full of deadly explosives, you are going to have limited success at best. But that's what many conventional approaches to stress and panic do. Some therapies *can* painstakingly cure panic this way; for instance, exposure with response prevention, which is a treatment I did in the old days.

If I had seen Alicia in 2005, we would have started with one avoidant behavior where improvement would have made her life easier—say, going to the grocery store so she wasn't dependent on expensive delivery. She would have imagined going to the store while taking steps to calm her nervous system through breathing, positive thoughts, or relaxation. After several sessions, we would trek out to the grocery store together, tracking her stress level and trying to keep her calm.

Each situation Alicia feared would have taken about twelve sessions to treat. Her extensive list of landmines might have taken over a year in therapy, with me crossing my fingers the whole time that no new landmines had to be added to the list. Also, she might have developed a dependence on Xanax, so we would have had to add more treatment to address that. And, it was always possible that after all that time in treatment, Alicia would still be coping with some degree of panic and avoidance. Meanwhile, months and years of her career, her life, and her potential would slip through her fingers.

With such tedious, unreliable treatment options to choose from, I can understand why, for decades now, many physicians have just thrown up their hands and written prescriptions. If their oath was to do no harm, relief through medication might have seemed like a better alternative.

In the past, treating chronic stress was like being in a leaky, water-logged boat while it rained. All we had was a coffee mug to bail out as much water as possible to stay afloat. There was no way to plug up the holes and paddle to sunny skies. Our best options were medication and treatments that were often not powerful enough to get rid of the problem entirely.

Today we have buckets and plugs for the holes, but we need to seek information and demand access to new options, especially for people like Alicia whose ships are sinking while they try to cope and manage chronic stress.

Fortunately, Alicia came to me in 2016, so I had some effective buckets to help bail out her boat. These were EMDR, cranial electrotherapy stimulation, and a home program of bilateral stimulation. (More on these and other ways I treat patients with chronic stress later.)

Want to guess the number of sessions until we brought her to zero panic attacks? Fifteen total. Not 120, not 85, but fifteen. She's now in a graduate school program she was previously too fearful to apply for and maintaining a healthy relationship. As for those landmines causing the explosions of panic? Gone.

Sure, Alicia still has stress in her life. Zero stress is unrealistic for any of us based on how our nervous systems are wired. But zero panic attacks, yes! **There *is* a cure for the unnecessary, excess stress response and anxiety that isn't serving us.** And now that you know there is a cure, I doubt that mere coping will still seem like the best option.

Changing Cope to Cure

I take issue with the way we talk about the need to "cope" with stress. Coping means you have a strategy for how to mitigate something bad that you assume is inevitable. It's a natural piece of the fight-or-flight response, but excess stress and anxiety can amplify a healthy coping strategy into to a full-blown, often debilitating avoidance response (sometimes, as in Alicia's case, accompanied by panic attacks).

Unfortunately, because too many doctors still believe there is no cure for these extreme reactions, they focus their treatments on coping with, instead of eliminating, excess stress. The result is that a mind-boggling number of Americans are stuck medicating their fear of tripping an adrenaline-fueled fight-or-flight landmine.

Change is slow in a big system. I even sometimes get resistance from therapists in training when I tell them we can fix a five-year-old's fear of the dark with twenty minutes of EMDR therapy versus twelve sessions of cognitive behavioral therapy (CBT). Even when see the research for themselves, their initial excitement at a cure is quickly followed by fear—how they are going to stay in business if curing can really be that fast? I remind them that if they do great work, word will spread, business will grow, and they can feel proud of helping patients in the most efficient ways possible. I'd say that's a better business model.

It's time to show you the difference some of these relatively new but highly effective treatments can make, but first, let me summarize some of the key points about how we think about stress and what we know about how it works.

It's Not Your Fault

Unfortunately, it's the patients who suffer when practitioners doubt the cure. Besides the heavy physical toll of medication and long-term chronic stress response, there is also an emotional toll in the form of self-blame. When it comes to stress many of us believe it's all in our minds, and that we should be able to control it ourselves, but cannot. We see stress as a sign of personal weakness. Time and time again, "I am a total stress case," is a self-condemnation, assuming our lack of control over our biology and current ways of being are somehow our fault.

You're Not Alone

Social media doesn't help us gain perspective. We compare our blooper reel to everyone else's highlight reels when we see images of happy, smiling friends and assume that, unlike us, they are stress-free and ecstatic in their lives. I'm not suggesting that we should add more negativity to social media by filling it with the worst versions of ourselves instead, but it's worth remembering that everyone does what everyone does: we only post the pretty stuff.

From the outside, people might make the stress-free and ecstatic assumption about me, for example. Meanwhile, my life is far from a fairy tale. I live alone with my two children and balancing can seem downright impossible on some days. One night, I was so exhausted that I literally cried when I saw we were out of milk. I had no physical or mental reserves to be able to pull off a simple trip to the grocery store with my six- and eight-year-olds that evening. Everyone has these hidden struggles we don't see—or post ourselves—on social media.

If you are stressed and overwhelmed, you are far from alone. After working with thousands of people over the years, I can tell you how the real blooper reels compare to social media. Stress is, unfortunately, a collective national condition.

You Aren't Broken

The fact that you have stress does not mean that you are broken, nor is it a life sentence. Stress is not a static condition like height or weight. It fluctuates in milliseconds via your autonomic system and largely without your conscious control. The particular way stress shows up in your system can be changed, but probably not in the ways you've been told. Until now you've probably been unaware of how to change stress and have either tried methods that worked a little or not at all. Until now, you probably didn't even know you could help yourself.

Temporarily Under the Weather

If I have the flu, it would be crazy for me to think I'd have to cope with the flu forever. Both my doctor and I would assume my immune system could fight it off, and I would get expect to get better. But we assume mental diagnoses are permanent in part because we have not understood their physical mechanisms the same way we understand how our immune systems fight off disease. We aren't thinking of things like panic or anxiety or stress as physical ailments, which they absolutely are, and that means we can measure and create treatments for their physical causes. I can see the level of cortisol (a hormone that the body produces under stress) spike in someone who is stressed out just the same way I can see a cancer cell in a petri dish. Stress is definitely physical, not just mental. It's time we think about it right.

Stress Response Is Designed to Lock Itself In

If you get stressed about something once, your brain will unconsciously imprint that response and trigger the stress switch again in similar situations in the future. That's how our brain keeps us alive—by learning how to avoid real threats of danger. However, when this natural response goes into a frequent, over-reactive state of fight-or-flight, like in Alicia's case, our lizard brain tells us to avoid daily activities and trips panic when it's unnecessary. This keeps happening until we un-trip those wires and get our nervous system back on track.

Badge of Honor

While many people add self-blame to their stress experience, at the other end of a variety of maladaptations to chronic stress, a portion of people have the opposite issue, Some people turn what should be seen as a problem to be solved into a badge of honor. Once a person lives in a problem for long enough, they begin to take ownership of it. When a medical problem is labeled chronic it becomes an accepted condition of life. In some cases, as a way of controlling the uncontrollable, many individuals will even embrace their condition.

For these people, stress has become less of a fault, and more of a character trait, direct evidence of how they're hard working, productive, valuable members of society. "If I'm stressed, with demands being placed on my time and energy," the reasoning goes, "I'm obviously important." Excess stress, they'll tell anyone who will listen, is part of the human condition. It's normal. If you're not stressed, you're doing something wrong. You're lazy, you're not working hard enough, and you're not good enough. Life is stressful; therefore you *should* be stressed.

Stress Is Not a Productivity Hack

The people who are telling you that stress is a part of life you should just learn to live with are denying a brutal health truth: excess stress is bad. Really, really bad. So bad that it's ruining your life and health before it quietly kills you. You might think you're managing it, but you are likely not. It is managing you—every part of you, every hour of every day, all the time. The longer you let it run rampant, unchecked, spilling its toxic mercury droplets into every cell of your body and every area of your life, the more it owns you. This is not something to strive for, and certainly nothing to be proud of. Yet, tragically, the badge of honor mentality has become a universal attitude about productivity in our culture.

When I worked at startup companies before I got my doctorate degree there was actually a bed in one of our offices that employees could use when they pulled all-nighters or were too exhausted to continue working. Although it was presented as a perk, the unintended message was, "You should be working so hard and be so stressed out and sleep deprived that if you don't fall down in a frazzled unconscious wreck onto the bed at least once every day, you're not doing your job." This is not productivity, people, this is insanity! Yet so many people are falling for it, and embracing it as a reality of work today.

Now, some good news. Ensuring a good outcome doesn't require more work. It doesn't require hardship. It requires easing into your work, and then a process of letting go. We need to uncouple the idea of working hard from blood, sweat, tears, and stress. Having a lot to do and being extremely stressed out about it are actually two separate things, but we often combine them and confuse them. Only when people finally de-stress do they fully realize how incredibly inefficient their stress has made them. Stress creates inefficiency in productivity because it is distracting and leads to poor communication, poor decision-making, and poor quality of work.

If I'm reading and can't focus because my brain is cycling with ten other things I have to do, I may think I'm being productive, but I won't comprehend it. Stress makes us repeat things. It makes us question things that don't need to be questioned. It makes us ponder things that don't need to be pondered, which actually distracts from our ability to just be present and do what we need to do.

Today's stressed out, overworked workers would make terrible farmers. After planting on soil for a period of time, agricultural farmers have to let the soil lay dormant for a little while before they replant. Otherwise the nutrients get so depleted that the soil becomes infertile. These farmers know that there are times when the highest and best use of their land is to replenish itself, to rest.

Off the farm, we have people on autopilot, working around the clock, burning enough midnight oil to ignite the whole planet, all the while thinking they're being productive. But they're not efficient, and in many cases they're barely conscious or functional. They're like a short-circuiting Energizer bunny, powered by a battery of caffeine and adrenaline from the stress of a completely unregulated adrenal system. They don't allow for any replenishment—and it's killing them slowly.

So let's say for the sake of argument that you're one of these people who have bought into the lie that not only is stress inevitable, it's a badge of honor. You have a giant S on your back for workplace superhero: your brain and body are running on empty, your nerve endings are fried, and you're constantly hanging on by a thread until that next deadline, break, or whichever other temporary finish lines you've drawn in your life.

Suddenly you're faced with a brand new trauma—your child gets hurt at school, an unexpected large bill arrives in the mail, a parent becomes ill, the rug gets pulled out from under a major project at work. How well do you think you will handle this new majorly stressful situation—mentally, physically, and emotionally? Most likely, not very well. Because the conditions caused by your overactive stress switch have weakened your defenses over time, this new event is likely to create an exaggerated stress response. In other words, you'll get WAY more stressed out and overwhelmed by it than you would if you were running on a full tank of gas. Because you have allowed yourself to go without enough sleep, food, or exercise, and stayed mentally stressed from overworking yourself for so long, you'll be a dried out pile of half-dead hay, just waiting for a lit match.

Does this sound like a state of physical, mental, and emotional being to be proud of? Denial—whether as a form of self-blame or a form of misplaced pride, is not the solution to chronic stress. And habitually perpetuating the cycle just isn't worth it.

Curing

If you knew that the only thing standing in the way of your full life's potential, all your personal and professional goals, was curable, would you take the cure? Surprisingly enough, many people would not.

These are people who have found a benefit in being impaired in some way. Sometimes it's better to not try than to try and fail. It's called self-handicapping. This means tossing up obstacles between you and success, so that when you fail, you get to blame the obstacles instead of your own skills and abilities. It's largely unconscious, but most of us are actually afraid of having no excuse, because that would me that we have no choice but to live up to our potential. Self-handicapping is a convenient mental mechanism to keep that from happening. If my back hurts, I can't do this...If I'm stressed out, I can't do that...If I didn't study, I have an excuse to fail the test...and the list goes on.

Clinging to the paradigm that chronic stress can only be coped with but never cured can be conveniently self-handicapping. The symptoms, constant treatments, and burden of having a chronic condition can seem like legitimate reasons to live safely within the confines of our comfort zones. Like a dog with an invisible leash, the responsibility that comes with coping with an incurable disease yanks us back whenever we stray too far.

And for most Americans, this is perfectly acceptable and normal; we've even built an entire language around the comforting idea that since there's nothing that can be done, we might as well find a way to live with it. To completely cure an incurable condition would require a total rewrite of our belief system.

In the case of cancer, they never say "cure," only "in remission," because it might come back. With alcoholism, people aren't "cured," they are perpetually "in recovery." We are terrified to think of saying once something is licked it will never occur again.

Think for a moment of how your life would change if all the unnecessary excess stress that is keeping you sick and holding you back from your goals just vanished. Most people aren't even aware of how much their excess stress is holding them back in life. For me, I wasn't just being held back—I was slowly dying.

My Stress Story

At twenty-seven I was *stressed*. My allergies were so severe that I would break out into hives every day. I had eczema rashes covering so much of my body that I avoided exercise because sweating was so painful that I would start crying. My body was so inflamed I felt like scratching my skin off most days. Once I allowed myself to do it, I would rub my face so vigorously that it swelled up. When I went to the ER, they brought in a team of residents to observe me because my case was apparently incredibly medically interesting.

To outsiders, I had a charmed life: my boyfriend was a Harvard-trained doctor trying to be supportive, but he was so caught up in his own career he only made me worry more about my condition by smothering me with all the diagnostic possibilities and suggesting every treatment under the sun. Obsessive and stressed himself, he was fearful of all of the possible side effects of topical ointments, but managed to convince to try an experimental drug that I was actually allergic to, which made things worse.

I was depressed, stressed, and working sixty hours a week plus a two-and-half-hour daily commute to a business development job at a startup company in Los Angeles that I knew wasn't aligned with my true calling. I knew I had to make a change, but had no idea where to begin. My stress switch was almost perpetually in the on position—I was operating in survival mode.

My doctor put me on an antidepressant and steroids, which helped a bit but caused me to gain 20 pounds, which then triggered my teenage body image issues to resurface. I became more depressed and self-deprecating than ever, and felt like my life was slipping away.

When my cat exacerbated my allergies, I adopted her to a family friend. Eating any fermented foods would cause me to break out in hives. I had to leave several work functions because my ears would get hot and red. I became used to the idea that this was going to be my life forever—overweight, sick, and stressed in the rat race of L.A. And to the outside world, it looked like I had a great job and a great boyfriend, and life was good.

Firmly entrenched in the misery of my world, I had no idea how immersed I was in the cascade of stress and disease. Finally, one night on the phone my mother gave me perspective. In tears, she quietly said, "Amy, you don't even sound like YOU. There's no joy in your voice. You're so far from who you are. Something needs to change."

Her sadness for me sent my mind working frantically, trying to remember my life before this horrifying chapter, but all I saw was the infinite darkness in front of me. I couldn't even remember happiness at the time because I was struggling so badly. A fish doesn't know it's swimming in water because water is all it knows! I was swimming in a sea of stress and ill health, and I was so caught up in the muck, I had no idea I used to feel differently.

I was in a tunnel and couldn't see the light. I had to learn to trust that the tunnel was not infinite. How long it was and how long I stayed in it depended on me. Looking back, I now realize this was the beginning of the paradigm shift I'm now introducing to you. I made the shift from coping with chronic stress—from believing that we have no other choice—to finding a cure.

Short-circuiting Stress

As a result of my personal paradigm shift, I invented TouchPoints, which are award-winning neuroscience technology wearables that can physically short-circuit your body's stress response. At the heart of the TouchPoints devices is something called bilateral stimulation, and they are based on the same treatments I've delivered to patients in my clinics for years.

Bilateral stimulation in tactile form has been used in doctors' and therapists' offices for over thirty years as part of EMDR therapy to treat chronic stress, PTSD, and other conditions.

My published research as a neuropsychologist has shown that bilateral stimulation technology has a safe and generalized response in significantly lowering the stress switch. A study of 1,109 subjects documented an average sixty-two percent stress reduction in thirty seconds.[11]

These revelatory results were even better than we hoped, and I realized that, with TouchPoints, we have discovered a global stress hack, accessible to everyone, that can be used safely anytime and anywhere, outside of doctors' offices. The genius of TouchPoints is that, unlike needing to make a therapy appointment, they provide stress relief anytime and anywhere and, ironically, for the approximate cost of one therapy session! This gives unlimited access to every man, woman, and child anywhere in the world. Imagine what widespread use can accomplish.

TouchPoints work because, as you learned earlier, stress originates in sensory information processing by the salience network. When your senses deliver information that your salience network interprets as trouble, it flips your stress switch on. TouchPoints, however, give it a different sensory input, essentially persuading the salience network to change its mind and dim the switch. It's important to note that once your stress switch reaches a certain point, you can't "dim it" with your thoughts, yoga, listening to soft music, or by talking yourself out of being stressed. Your stress switch needs a specific sensory input to dim down and turn off, one that TouchPoints are specifically engineered to create. They seem to cause your salience network to make a different decision faster and more effectively than other methods of "stress relief."

TouchPoints can also lower your stress baseline—the point on the stress dimmer switch where your body becomes triggered and stress escalates from mild to moderate, and then from moderate to severe. I believe each time you use TouchPoints when you're stressed, new neural pathways are created in your brain, essentially rewriting how you respond to stress. Over time, a new, calmer baseline can result.

Creating TouchPoints has allowed me to help total strangers using the same science I use to help countless patients in my clinics every day. By thinking differently and looking where other doctors, researchers, and practitioners were not looking, I advanced the science and technology of bilateral brain stimulation and made it more accessible to the public.

You'll get a clearer idea of how TouchPoints can physically hack stress as they pop up in stories and case studies throughout the book. For now, the most important thing you need to know is that with TouchPoints, my goal is to shift existing paradigms around the treatment of stress. And now, this book gives me the opportunity to help you shift your paradigm about stress, too!

Imagine if every single one of these statements were true:

- We can cure panic attacks by changing the nervous system's reactivity so that panic doesn't occur anymore—ever.

- We can cure PTSD: no more flashbacks, triggers, nightmares, or emotional reactivity—ever.

- We can cure excess stress—no more going into fight-or-flight, much less full-blown panic, when someone's life isn't in danger.

- We can cure stress-related avoidance—no more procrastination, underachievement, phobias, or social anxiety.

- We can prevent stress-related disorders from even starting.

I am asking you to believe that every one of these statements is possible. Better coping skills for stress should not be our goal. Coping as a goal implies the problem will be persistent in our lives and can't be changed. Together we can do better than cope. I believed that my stress could be cured, took action to make it true, and in the process, changed my own beliefs about stress. Because of that shift, I essentially came back from the dead, and I am rising up to meet my full potential as a human being. You can too. I'm here to tell you a better life is possible, and together you and I can work to achieve it.

Part II: Breakdown

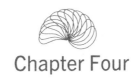

Chapter Four

HOW STRESS GETS IN YOUR WAY

Unchecked stress is like mercury in a pond that can ruin the entire ecosystem. Stress poisons our health and productivity, and then poisons our view of ourselves. Stress becomes the lens through which we see the world, and it can literally ruin our lives before it kills us.

Drops of Mercury

Stress is like mercury in a pond. As each shimmering, silver drop of mercury slips beneath the water's surface, it splits apart over and over into smaller droplets, eventually infiltrating and becoming one with every drop of water in the pond. One single drop of mercury can poison an entire pond. That's how excess stress works in your body.

The distinction you're going to learn now is that excess stress is never "just stress," or isolated to one area of your body, or even one area of your life. Excess stress affects your entire being. It touches every single cell of your body.

There is a distinction between normal stress and pond-poisoning excess stress. Some stress has a positive role. We need a little bit of stress to create energy for some activities. Mild amounts of stress can motivate us to make changes, such as eating healthier if we want to avoid being overweight, or working for an extra hour with increased focus if we want to finish a project before a deadline. The key word here is mild; go beyond mild and performance starts to worsen instead of improve.

Excess stress exists above and beyond that sort of normal, healthy mild stress. Simply put: excess stress is usually unnecessary for your survival, and that's the kind you want to lessen. So when I talk about stress in this book, I'm talking about excess stress.

Physically, excess stress is the equivalent of that mercury in the pond. The stress switch sets off a cascade of changes that inflames the body and shuts down adaptive processes in the brain, while cortisol, adrenaline, and other chemicals spread like slippery droplets of mercury, leaving no part of us untouched. When our stress hormones and chemicals hit their peak from the stimuli overload, they inflame our bodies, affecting every single cell. Excess stress is killing us slowly. This section of the book will reveal how and where it's happening.

Breaking It Down

The chapters in this section present the surprising ways stress affects your mind, body, and life. I say surprising because when you think of stress, you probably know the common symptoms associated with stress—like trouble sleeping, cravings, headaches, high blood pressure, and the overall mental strain that makes you throw up your hands and declare, "I'm so stressed!"

However, the immediate and long-term manifestations of stress spread far beyond that list of common symptoms, because experiencing stress creates immediate physical changes in your brain and body that dictate your behavior, your emotions, your ability to communicate, and how you react to the world.

That's why I'm covering some of the most common problems that people struggle with when they seek help from me: avoidance, performance issues, trouble connecting with others, selfishness, impulsivity, pessimism, sleep, and PTSD. People are frequently surprised to find out that the issues on the list can be a direct result of stress.

How these stress struggles translate to real life varies, but there are common themes. Stressed couples can become locked into a pattern of selfishness and conflict, losing the ability to empathize with their partners. Stressed executives become paralyzed in negative thinking and pessimism, unable to move their companies or their lives forward. Stressed managers procrastinate and avoid problems to the point of losing their jobs. Stressed mothers can't stop obsessive thoughts about all of their responsibilities and then can't fall asleep. Stressed teens start behavioral or chemical addictions. This list goes on and on and on... Most people don't recognize stress as the culprit behind these behaviors. They instead categorize these issues as isolated problems of an unknown origin, and often assume they can't be solved. As when mercury has poisoned a pond, they're able to see each fish and rock and identify individual problems, but they fail to see the poison that has infiltrated the entire body of water.

The bad news here is that unchecked stress begets more stress. When the entire pond is affected, when excess stress is poisoning every cell in your body, the number and intensity of events that stress you out in life shoots up, along with the time it takes you to recover from those events. When your body is stressed, something that you'd likely shake off as a bad day can escalate into a physical and emotional pit of molasses, keeping you stuck in what might otherwise have been a brief blip on your life radar.

Now for some good news—the inverse is also true. Calm begets more calm. How? Well, for starters, your stress level in any moment affects how you process new information received in that moment. For example, we had a huge swarm of bees this year outside of my house, and I hadn't figured out what to do with them yet, because I didn't want to kill them. Nonetheless, I realized that my children, ages nine and ten, were going to notice the thousand or so bees buzzing just under the roof of our two-story home, and that might create some serious anxiety, especially if they stumbled upon them unexpectedly.

So what's a neuropsychologist mom do with situations like this to avoid activating their fight-or-flight mechanism and thus thwart a potential future phobia of bees? I put TouchPoints in their hands and said, "Hey, come here you guys, I want you to look at something."

Then, we all walked out together to look at the bee swarm as the TouchPoints buzzed in my children's hands, providing bilateral brain stimulation that dramatically reduced their stress levels in that critical moment.

As we approached the swarm, I reassured them: "These are not the Africanized killer bees, so it's okay to look from a distance and notice how cool it is that they are all in this big honeycomb."

I added for good measure, "Don't worry, I am going to take care of them soon, but for now, we are going to avoid this side of the house, just in case. It would be OK if you got stung, but it's not pleasant, so we're going to take some precautions."

Still holding their TouchPoints, both children looked at me calmly and said, "Okay."

Your existing stress level determines how you receive and process information in the moment. This is great news if you are calm, and your brain is actively processing new information. However, if your baseline is a stressed state, the reactivity of situations like these will be worse, and the stress cycle will perpetuate itself. Had I seen the bees, run into the house screaming, and triggered everyone's fight-or-flight mechanisms, we would have all suffered, and my children and even I may have started avoiding pools, the outdoors, or become preoccupied about bees in the future, because the fear could have been locked into our fear/memory systems. Using TouchPoints in that moment allowed me to prevent all that. We were able to move on with our day and our lives because the technology allowed them to be calm to process the information. (As a side note, those bees had created about forty pounds of honeycomb in my attic, and we were able to save 25,000 of them!)

Bad Medicine

Let's say I didn't have TouchPoints, and one of my children saw the bees, got stung, and then developed a phobia of bees. If I took them to a psychiatrist, the doctor might have prescribed an anti-anxiety medication for them. The medicine wouldn't have cured the phobia, but it would have given my son a remedy for his stress switch if he saw a bee in the future or his stress switched turned on at the thought of a bee. This isn't necessarily a bad course of action, if the doctor's aim is to treat the acute stress in these situations—it's just that temporarily lowering stress with pharmacology often leaves the underlying problem, well, still a problem.

At this point you might be wondering, "If doctors know that stress can poison our entire mind and body and negatively affect us in so many ways, why don't they go right to the source and eliminate the cause of excess stress, rather than temporarily blocking the symptoms of stress with chemicals that have negative side effects? Why aren't they addressing the root cause?"

This is a perfectly sensible question, especially in light of the parade of prescriptions filing into pharmacies on a regular basis to treat what, in many cases, are symptoms of underlying stress.

It's not that doctors don't know the effects of excess stress and the neurology of stress. They know stress is autonomic, but they are not looking at solutions that address the salience network's ability to switch the stress switch on and off.

They see the effects of the mercury just fine too. They medicate the high blood pressure, operate on chronic back pain that has no apparent physical cause, send scopes down the gastrointestinal tracts of children with chronic stomach problems, prescribe more and more anti-anxiety medications to patients who aren't seeing relief of their symptoms. I can't fault them for trying the best they can, based on their point of view of the problem.

Every day they send teams of different kinds of researchers into the pond to find out what's poisoning it. One team looks at the rocks, one looks at the fish, and another looks at the algae. They look at each individual piece of the pond and try to figure out how to make it thrive again. Then, together, they come up with an incredibly complex treatment to clean up the rocks, resuscitate the dying fish, and make the algae resume growing.

But nobody takes a step back, looks at the pond, and says, "Why don't we remove that mercury that's poisoning everything and then come up with a solution to undo the damage?"

When I was in my twenties, and excess stress had caused my entire body to become inflamed, my doctor suggested a turbinectomy, a surgery in which nasal tissue is removed to improve breathing. I reluctantly complied. But my body stayed inflamed, and my allergies were worse than ever. When I went back to my doctor, he recommended more surgery. He wanted to keep cleaning rocks, fertilizing algae, and doing CPR on fish. Meanwhile, the mercury (my excess stress) was destroying me.

Needless to say, I went in a different direction. I treated my stress. When I went back to that doctor, he examined my nasal passages with amazement and said, "This is looking great! What have you been doing?" I told him: exercise, therapy, PTSD treatment, and learning how to be happy, among other things.

He smiled the way you smile at a child when they misunderstand an adult topic of conversation and said, "No, I meant, what *medications* did you take?"

I replied, "None."

I can only assume he went back to examining the rocks, fish, and algae, thinking I was at best, a statistical anomaly and at worst, completely unbelievable. I think he thought I was certifiably nuts or, at the very least, lying to him.

How is it logical for us to still be looking at this pond where mercury (stress) has been introduced into the ecosystem (the body) and naively saying, "Oh my gosh, this is so weird. The algae aren't healthy, the fish aren't healthy, the fauna aren't growing, and the rocks lining the shores aren't growing moss like they should. And when the animals drink from the pond, they get sick, too. What a coincidence that all these problems occur!"

At some point, someone has to seek to connect the dots and identify a common cause. It would only be a matter of time until they would shout, "It's the mercury! Stop looking at each individual thing, stop analyzing the rocks, stop examining the fish, it's the mercury!"

If we start with the mercury of stress, learn how it's getting into the pond, and stop the pollution before it begins, the problems it causes will be solved. The fish will get better, the algae will get better, the moss will get better, the plants will get better—everything will get better if we address the mercury.

Untreated excess stress equates to ruined relationships, lost jobs, emotional pain, and unresolved physical conditions like migraines, allergies, and Crohn's disease. As scientists, we need to stop looking at individual symptoms under a microscope and trying to fix them one by one. In the pond, it's the mercury. And in the human condition, it's the untreated stress. The good news is we know stress is the cause—we've found the answer.

Now that we have it, we no longer have to be running around exhausting ourselves looking for the perfect blend of B6s and B12s and amino acids and essential oils and theories from biohackers. We know that stress leads to inflammation, which leads to ill health, which leads to poor behavior, which leads to irritability, which leads to you being distracted, which leads to you avoiding things that you like, which leads to you not being your best, which leads to you narrowing your world down, which leads to you not living at *your* full potential. There is no need whatsoever to study the minutiae in the pond for fifty more years and then end up with the same pond at the end.

I'm asking the teams of scientists to pull back, get out of the pond, and stop over-complicating everything. We've over-complicated diagnoses and even worse, treatments. We're not helping people by doing this. We're getting in the way of the cure and in doing so, leaving people to suffer from the effects of stress. We're leaving them to fall short of their full human potential.

Your Full Potential

I did not understand all of this when I started creating TouchPoints. At first, I only had what my patients using our prototypes and their EEG data were showing me. But then, suddenly, I was going through a divorce, and excess stress was routinely blocking any sort of clear, rational thought (those of you who have gone through a divorce know what I mean). When I started using TouchPoints to reduce my own stress, I was able to experience firsthand what they can do.

Now I had this invention that took away my excess stress nearly instantly. On even the worst days, I could be patient, communicate clearly, think more rationally, and they helped me be more productive. It wasn't just in my head either; there were real changes in my brain. As I documented the effects of TouchPoints, electroencephalograms (EEGs) of my brain showed improved electrical activity in the areas that are associated with stress and with the ability to think positively rather than negatively. As my team continued developing the TouchPoints technology, the list of subjective and objective results that I experienced whenever I used them kept growing. And that is when I truly saw for myself all the different areas of my body and life that stress had touched... like mercury in a pond. I really had no idea how much stress had taken from me, until I removed it.

It has been a serendipitous journey, from my own debilitating stress-triggered illness, a PhD in Neuropsychology, the invention of TouchPoints, and finally, the removal of my own excess stress, to help me get out of my own way enough to see the true and far-reaching effects of stress. In the meantime, every day that I was held captive by stress was a day wasted not reaching my full potential. If I hadn't gotten out of my own way by removing my stress, I would not be where I am today—not even close. You certainly would not be reading this book right now.

Stress will hold you back from reaching your full potential in life. Successes are eluding you because of the stress that is disconnecting you from all you are capable of being. Where would you be in life without stress? How far could you go without the excess stress that you think you need or you think is normal and unavoidable?

Stress takes you out of a state of calm by creating an inflamed, uncomfortable, out-of-sync body, leading to pain, cravings, and other problems. With physical distress comes poor performance, decreased focus, thoughtlessness, and disconnectedness, all of which increase the likelihood of becoming selfish, angry, and hurtful to others. This means that stress affects not only your own quality of life but also how you treat others. It contributes to a fundamental understanding of who you are within society.

When a state of distress and disconnect is left unchecked, it will ultimately do far more than cause physical and emotional distress in the moment. Unaddressed stress is a profound problem that, like mercury in a pond, first poisons our health and our daily lives, and then, when seen as incurable, poisons our very identity and view of ourselves. Stress becomes the lens through which we see the world and ourselves. In a sense, it becomes our own personal operations and ethics manual. And this affects every single person in our lives, whether we're willing to acknowledge it or not.

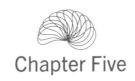

Chapter Five

STORM WITHIN THE CALM

No matter what is happening outside of you, stress can rage like a storm inside. No one looks out the window and sees a tornado whipping up shrubs, tearing off rooftops, swirling dust violently into a vortex, and says "everything is fine here, let's go swimming." So why do we ignore the storm within? The answer is that we don't always sense the storm at all.

When life is good but they're still stressed, people become frustrated. They see the apparent calm of a good life outside, and don't understand that within that calm, a storm can still roar. People tend to believe that if their current external reality is generally good, their internal reality should match it. But it won't matter how you adjust external circumstances in an attempt to relieve stress; if you don't regulate your brain and your nervous system to be calm, you will not feel calm. As a therapist and researcher, it's my job to identify and treat the storm within the calm.

Anne

Forty-five year-old Anne came to me to find out why she was experiencing significant stress and anxiety, hyper-vigilance, and fear when her current life "was great." In her mind, her symptoms made no sense, because she had a nice husband, wonderful children, financial security, a fulfilling career, and felt like she should be grateful and happy. But she wasn't. Her stress symptoms approached the level of PTSD.

Although her adult life was "great," her childhood had been a much different story. Anne had grown up in the foster care system, and although her foster family had been loving and kind, the first five years of her life were incredibly chaotic. Anne had learned about the chaos secondhand, and like most people, she thought if she didn't remember it, it shouldn't be affecting her.

As Anne told me, "I know my life had been chaotic because of what people have told me, but I don't remember it. I have a college degree, a nice husband, and great children. I should feel really happy and calm, not be having panic attacks and anxiety."

It is common thinking that conscious memory dictates whether or not we should be stressed out or be affected by events. Our hippocampus, which is a very important brain area for learning and memory, isn't fully online at a young age, and most people have very few conscious memories before around age four. But you don't need memories to be traumatized or to remember stress, because your body encodes it anyway. Periods of extreme stress that occur while brain functions are still developing can cause the brain to develop differently, so the damage is done regardless of whether or not you remember it.

Even in the absence of conscious memories, the brain can still match sensory triggers to what happened before age four, and neglect, abuse, and a lack of parental bonding in those early years can shape the brain to be hyper-sensitive and over-reactive to stress. Children who were neglected have even been shown to have lower IQs than those who were nurtured.

So it really didn't matter neurologically if Anne remembered the early trauma and neglect or not. According to child psychiatrist Bruce Perry, "Children aren't resilient, they are malleable."[12] Your brain and body absolutely log early trauma and make them a part of your permanent record. Anne's nervous system was hard-wired to be over-reactive and stressed.

Here is what Anne's brain and body had recorded when she was a child. Her biological mother was a prostitute, so she and Anne were constantly relocating to different homes, apartments, and they even lived in mom's car for a while. Mom had multiple boyfriends, with whom she would leave Anne when she went to work at a variety of jobs. Mom was also drug-addicted and eventually lost custody, which is why Anne was placed in the foster care system.

In her adult life, even though Anne had been successful in layering on the good—making good choices and surrounding herself with wonderful people—her stress system remained hard-wired to be overactive. All the good choices in the world were not going to be strong enough to undo that early-age wiring. Stress was literally embedded in her nervous system, brain structure, and brain function.

We've talked about how the fear, anxiety, and stress systems are autonomic. Because these involuntary systems are functional at birth even while other functions like conscious memories are not, as a small child, Anne's brain was in a state of chaos and even terror as a result of not having her basic needs met—like not being soothed when she needed soothing, lacking shelter and safety, not having regular sleep and wake cycles, and possibly even being physically abused or neglected. Consequently, her brain developed abnormally and in a way that made it over-reactive as an adult. Therefore, no matter what she did, she could not shake these feelings of fear, hyper-vigilance and internal chaos.

Nervous System Memories

Anne is the definition of the storm within the calm. Even without childhood trauma, people can embody the storm within the calm. Do you know anyone who to escapes to a beach to listen to the relaxing sounds of waves lapping gently on the shore under a clear blue sky? And the whole time, their inner dialogue chatters away about the hundreds of emails they'll be coming back to, the big company project coming apart at the seams because of interoffice politics, their recent break-up and all the ugly words exchanged, and everything else stressing them out in their regular life? You can tell this person that they can lie on that beach all they want, but as long their nervous system is shorting out like a downed wire flopping around on the road after a hurricane, there's no way that some sunshine and a margarita is getting through to stop it. It's not physically possible. No matter how powerful the calm, the storm is still raging. No matter how you adjust external circumstances to relieve stress, if you don't regulate your brain and your nervous system to be calm, you will not feel calm.

Another example from my clinic is the parent with a child experiencing general anxiety who tells me, "Johnny is so stressed out, we think we're going to change schools." Now, there are instances where an external situation such as an inappropriate environment is causing extreme anxiety, but in the case of a child who is anxious in *most* situations, changing one environment is usually not going to help.

In these cases, I refocus the conversation to teach the parents about the storm within the calm. They could put Johnny in the most perfect school ever, but wherever Johnny goes, there Johnny is, and the storm within the calm will still be there with him. It is impossible to run away from your own nervous system.

Before people make drastic external changes in their lives, I prompt them to make internal changes first, and then decide if they want to disrupt things on a larger scale. I've seen families move across a state, and switch their children's schools three times. People ditch romantic partners and partners over and over and over and some move across the world to new countries, all with the hopes that "things will be different this time." All of them are trying to outrun what they don't realize is a raging internal storm. Wherever we go, there we are. If we don't attend to the involuntary, autonomic processes that are causing stress and anxiety, then no matter how we change our external circumstances, it's not going to be the magic trick we think it will. Changing someone's circumstances can change their state of mind only if they're capable of calm.

For Anne, and for others like her, no amount of perfection in her external environment was going to change her brain enough. At the Serin Center clinics, we have developed a portfolio of treatments for the root causes of over-reactive stress that reduce the storm within the calm. They include EMDR, which is a psychotherapy treatment that heals the results of traumatic life experiences; neurofeedback, which uses an electroencephalogram to map brain function in real time so the therapist and patient can regulate it with operant conditioning; and my TouchPoints technology.

Anne completed a course of EMDR and neurofeedback, and used TouchPoints at home for a half-hour a day and five minutes prior to sleep each night. We did all this in order to still her internal storm and regulate her brain so that her internal state was in harmony with her external environment, and she could finally enjoy life.

Even though Anne's trauma was so early in her life, treatment was successful. However, early trauma is often more difficult to treat than trauma experienced as an adult. This is because the earlier and more pervasive the trauma was, the greater the number of neural connections which must be disrupted to reset the brain. Our therapy took about a year, which is quite a long time in comparison to many patients in my Serin Center clinics. Trauma patients usually reach all of their goals and reset maladaptive functioning in a few months by combining integrative treatments. But the earlier and more pervasive the trauma, and the longer the time elapsed until eventual treatment, the more extensive the treatment that will be required to solve the problems.

This is an important note in terms of how people heal: there is a direct correlation between the amount of elapsed time between trauma and treatment and the amount of time it will take to undo the effects of the trauma. If I see a child who has been abused or neglected, but there's no brain injury and he is now in a supportive environment, and I'm able treat him right afterwards, I can oftentimes undo most of the effects of the trauma. It is possible to reset his brain in a sense, erasing the emotional recording of traumatic incidents and preventing the fallout that will ensue if untreated.

What does it mean if, like Anne, you are experiencing signs of stress on a regular basis, but as far as you know or believe, you did not experience any past traumatic incidents? Remember that stress, including trauma, isn't defined by whether you think something should be upsetting from a logical point of view. There's no "should" in defining stress. The right question to ask is, "how did your brain interpret the experience?"

If you're showing signs of stress in the present and there is no imminent external threat, it is more than likely that something was recorded in your nervous system in the past. That doesn't mean you have repressed memories of physical or sexual abuse. That just means that something, somewhere along the way is affecting you. It doesn't have to have been earth-shattering or life-threatening. But it needs to be acknowledged. The what, where, why, and how of it doesn't need to be figured out—that all comes along with the healing. The bottom line is that if you can relate to what I'm saying, no matter how calm things are outside of you, the storm inside is real.

ACEs

In many cases, the storms are created in childhood, and are a result of Adverse Childhood Experiences, or ACEs, such as having grown up with someone who was severely depressed; having parents who divorced; having lived with someone who was verbally, sexually, or physically abusive; and/or having lived with someone with an active addiction. Children with chaotic upbringings such as Anne's, who were later adopted into stable, happy environments, frequently have the physical brain changes and signs of stress that cause their adopted parents to scratch their heads and ask, "Why is she stressed out? We've given her such a nice environment. She has everything she wants and is surrounded by love."

Well, unfortunately, the mercury (stress) from his or her early childhood chaos has already been disseminated into that child's pond; the information has already been recorded onto the nervous system and the brain has built hyper-connectivity and hyper-vigilance into the child's stress system. The brain itself has physically changed.

In research studies of children who have lived in orphanages, there is about a twenty-IQ point difference between these children and children who grow up with their biological families, in the absence of trauma. What's more, other studies have shown that the longer children stay in the orphanages, the lower their resulting IQ.[13,14]

Why is this? Orphanages are typically very stressful environments, with not enough nurturing to go around, and often little or no bonding happens. As a result, children's brains develop cognitive deficits, inadequate self-soothing mechanisms, and their stress switches became very overactive. Some of the most heartbreaking cases I've seen over the years in my clinics have been with children who were adopted from Russia, where orphanages are staffed in a particularly hands-off way. Their adoptive parents wonder how things could have turned out so poorly in their lives after all the nurturing they were able to provide once they adopted the child. Unfortunately, no one educated those well-meaning adoptive families about brain development in an orphanage setting and what can and cannot be undone.

Thank goodness, modern-day orphanages may be changing. One Russian study has shown that replacing a cold, unfeeling staff culture with warm, responsive caregiving improved physical growth, intellectual ability, social ability, and emotional regulation in the children during the study period.[15]

Early childhood trauma and neglect isn't confined to international orphanages. This is where the ACEs study comes into play. Between 1995 and 1997, Kaiser Permanente and the Centers for Disease Control and Prevention recruited participants for a well-documented study that demonstrated an association between ACEs and physical and mental problems throughout life, adverse health behaviors, and early death.[16,17] This was a landmark in research, because it showed that adverse childhood experiences are strongly related to poor physical health and mental disorders This is scientific proof that stress is not a "suck it up and get over it" mental problem to outwit. Stress changes us as organisms. We know that if we don't help individuals with ACEs to calm and soothe their nervous systems throughout their lifespan, they are going to experience social, emotional, and cognitive impairments, high-risk behaviors that are bad for their health, disease, disability, social problems, and even early death.

ACEs Assessment

The following is the standard ACEs questionnaire, adapted from the original ACEs study, which will give your ACEs score.[18] For each of the ten incidents described, give yourself a "1" if it happened to you. Feel free to take a few minutes now to stop and do the questionnaire, just so you understand what I'm referring to.

While you were growing up, during your first 18 years of life:

1. Did a parent or other adult in the household often...

Swear at you, insult you, put you down, or humiliate you?

OR

Act in a way that made you afraid that you might be physically hurt?

YES / NO   If yes, enter 1:

2. Did a parent or other adult in the household often...

Push, grab, slap, or throw something at you?

OR

Ever hit you so hard that you had marks or were injured?

YES / NO   If yes, enter 1:

3. Did an adult or person at least 5 years older than you ever...

Touch, fondle you or have you touch their body in a sexual way?

OR

Try to or actually have oral, anal, or vaginal sex with you?

YES / NO   If yes, enter 1:

4. Did you often feel that...

No one in your family loved you or thought you were important or special?

OR

Your family didn't look out for each other, feel close to each other, or support each other?

YES / NO   If yes, enter 1:

5. Did you often feel that...

You didn't have enough to eat, had to wear dirty clothes, and had no one to protect you?

OR

You parents were too drunk or high to take care of you or take you to the doctor if you needed it?

YES / NO   If yes, enter 1:

6. Were your parents ever separated or divorced?

YES / NO   If yes, enter 1:

7. Was your mother or stepmother:

Often pushed, grabbed, slapped, or had something thrown at her?

OR

Sometimes or often kicked, bitten, hit with a fist, or hit with something hard?

OR

Ever repeatedly hit over at least a few minutes or threatened with a gun or knife?

YES / NO   If yes, enter 1:

8. Did you ever live with anyone who was a problem drinker or alcoholic or who used street drugs?

YES / NO   If yes, enter 1:

_____

9. Was a household member depressed or mentally ill or did a household member attempt suicide?

YES / NO   If yes, enter 1:

_____

10. Did a household member go to prison?

YES / NO   If yes, enter 1:

_____

Now add up your "YES" answers. This is your ACEs Score.

I have an ACEs score of zero. I had an amazing childhood, and I am incredibly lucky. But as an adult, I chose for many years to be with a partner with an ACEs score of nine, and I saw first-hand the long-term effects on his life. He could not emotionally regulate himself, although he was very smart and had an advanced education. He tried his best to be a good person. Unfortunately, the structural changes in his brain caused by early and pervasive abuse created hyper-vigilance, personality problems, obesity, and depression, and he is now at high risk for health problems in the future. He had difficulty maintaining relationships and often extended his internal storm to create external storms as well. Most of us know people like this, and we watch them create unnecessary drama and suffering for others because they are suffering themselves.

Proactive, Early Treatment for ACEs

If we want to prevent the damage traumatized high-ACEs adults cause to themselves and others through addiction, anger, physical disease, violence, and underachievement, we need to help them as early as possible so their nervous systems and brains regulate throughout the development of their lifespan. When I see the outcomes of high ACEs scores in adults manifest in self-harm and harm to others, I can't help but shake my head in disbelief that we aren't doing more.

This is one of the reasons why I created TouchPoints. Children in the United States who have high ACEs scores may have access to therapy through state funding, but often times the therapy is led by interns and is done with modalities that don't alter things significantly. The usual modalities are like trying to empty out water in a sinking boat with a thimble instead of a bucket. Traumatized children need something that can regulate their nervous systems when they are outside of a therapist's office. We can't simply talk them out of their internal storms, and we can't just let this go and pretend there's not a problem.

To be effective with high-ACEs children, we have to bring their bodies back to homeostatic regulation and calm the nervous system as much as possible. If we do that, we have a chance of drastically improving their outcomes. A child with an ACES score of nine is at a 4,600 percent increased risk of developing COPD at some time in their life, and will have an average lifespan twenty years shorter than somebody with a low ACEs score. With early and correct treatment, we may be able to make that "9" child look like a "3" in terms of outcome. But we have to look at stress; we have to address the mercury in the pond. It is irresponsible to turn a blind eye to their behavioral problems, punish them or label them ADHD, and eventually funnel them into the juvenile court system. We can't just let these children go and see how far their unregulated nervous systems take them, often into addiction, crime, serious health problems, and early death.

The key to helping high-ACEs children have better futures is to re-regulate their nervous systems *as* they are developing—not take a wait-and-see approach or assume that trauma has to lead to all of these terrible outcomes. If we can intervene successfully, and I believe we can, we can change the entire outcome of someone's life.

114

We could really begin to bring the pond back to a healthy state, and actually remove some effects of that mercury. We may not be able to get rid of all of it, but with our new science and understanding of the threat response, we can deal with it effectively and make a significant impact.

ACEs Prevalence & Outcomes

Here's a closer look at the 1995 Kaiser Permanente ACES study. There were 17,337 total participants: seventy-five percent were Caucasian, the average age was fifty-seven, and seventy-five percent had attended college. All the participants had jobs and good health care. Twenty-eight percent had reported physical abuse, and twenty-one percent reported sexual abuse. Almost forty percent of the sample reported two or more ACEs, and 12.5 percent experienced four or more. ACEs occur in clusters, so if somebody has any ACEs at all (versus zero), they're more likely to have more than one. And as their number rises, it's likely to rise even more due to the clustering effect. Sixty-seven percent of study participants reported at least one adverse childhood experience, and of that group, eighty-seven percent reported at least one additional ACE. Think of the adage, "when it rains, it pours."

All of the ACEs were associated with high-risk behaviors such as smoking, alcohol and drug abuse, promiscuity, and severe obesity, as well as diseases like depression, heart disease, cancer, chronic lung disease, and an overall shorter lifespan. The more ACEs someone had, the higher the number and severity of high-risk behaviors and diseases they are likely to develop. Compared with an ACEs score of zero, a score of four was associated with a 700 percent increase in alcoholism, a doubled risk of cancer, and a four-fold increase in emphysema. An ACEs score above six equaled a 3,000 percent increase in attempted suicide.

The link between ACEs and high-risk behaviors like substance abuse and behavioral problems is probably less surprising than the link between ACEs and serious diseases like cancer, heart disease, and lung disease. But this link exists because disease is moderated by inflammation in the body, and inflammation is created by stress. If we ignore this link, we are missing the boat—one of many boats, as a matter of fact.

A different study by the Area Health Education Center of Washington State University found that students with an ACEs score of three or higher were three times as likely to experience academic failure, six times as likely to have behavioral problems, and five times as likely to have attendance problems. They also demonstrated problems trusting teachers and other adults, and had difficulty creating and maintaining relationships.[19, 20]

Why does stress result in misbehavior, poor adjustment, lower intelligence, and so many other problems? One theory is from Bruce S. McEwen. He coined the term *allostatic load* to describe the adaptive processes that maintain homeostasis during times of toxic stress by adjusting the body's production of adrenaline, cortisone, and other stress-mediating chemicals.[21] According to McEwen, these mediators of the stress response promote adaptation in the aftermath of acute stress, but they also contribute to allostatic overload: excessive wear and tear on the body and brain that results from being stressed out.

Allostatic overload is a short-term solution to acute stress, but it creates long-term problems (ACES outcomes). It follows that if we reduce the allostatic overload by helping the body to restore itself to homeostasis, over time we should be able to disrupt the negative physical and mental health outcomes from high ACEs scores. Enter the need for daily use of TouchPoints during a child's development, along with trauma-processing and other health behaviors, which I'll discuss later in the book.

Calm Waters

How do you calm the adult storm raging as a result of ACEs? For Anne and others with high ACEs scores, one of the most important things to do is process the trauma. By processing trauma, I don't mean that she had to simply remember the chaotic childhood she had forgotten. Processing trauma entails recalling the vivid or fragmented memories and the linked self-beliefs as a result, coupled with desensitization (a lowering of stress reactivity during recall). The two treatments recommended by the World Health Organization are EMDR therapy and trauma-focused CBT.[22] At the Serin Center clinics we primarily use EMDR because it tends to work faster. A typical EMDR session is similar to a talk therapy session: the patient sits in a comfortable office with a doctor or mental health counselor. Unlike talk therapy, however, the eight-phase EMDR process is systematic in identifying a current trigger that may link to past trauma, associated negative beliefs, localized stressful body sensations, rankings of degree of distress. The EMDR process also creates a future template of how and what the patient wants to feel and do once healed. The protocol includes check-ins by the therapist to determine how much the patient's ratings of distress are lowering in real time. Most of the active processing is non-verbal—which means talking about details of the trauma isn't necessary for healing. This is good news for young children who don't have words to describe things, for people who are too ashamed to discuss details of what they've done or experienced, and for our first responders and military who can't discuss classified information. For Anne, the ability to process trauma non-verbally was good news, because she couldn't remember specific traumas that occurred so early.

Despite Anne's lack of specific traumatic memories, the signs and symptoms of her high ACEs score were undeniable: She was anxious, hyper-vigilant, self-critical, panicked, prone to taking things personally, and had troubled sleep. Anne also tried hard to be perfect, which led her to create a great-looking life on the outside, while on the inside she felt very fragmented and had no ability to control her stress and anxiety.

In a series of attempts to treat the symptoms of her underlying problem in her teen and early adult years, Anne's doctors had prescribed several different antidepressants and anti-anxiety medications. She endured a lot of switching of these medications, which led to painful side effects and rebounding, accompanied by the emotional torment that nothing was working and she was still "bad." She developed feelings of inadequacy and eventually depression. When she became pregnant, she'd felt she had to choose between her unborn child's health and her own, and felt incredibly guilty that she had chosen to take medication when she was pregnant. Because of her unaddressed ACEs, her raging storm within the calm, Anne was put through hell and back—all over again.

It wasn't enough for Anne to talk about her feelings in therapy, or simply try to recall the abuse she'd forgotten. We needed to rebuild a better brain for Anne from the inside out; one that wasn't so hyper-sensitive to stimuli. We also needed a permanent solution, rather than processing only certain traumas and then having her come back in a year with a whole new list, because her brain would still be vulnerable to new situations becoming traumatic.

First, we used EMDR therapy to process the trauma, in conjunction with the following. In order to stabilize her brain functioning, Anne completed a course of neurofeedback and cranial electrical stimulation (CES),[23] implemented dietary changes and supplements, and used TouchPoints devices daily. That may seem like a lot, but many of those treatments could be done at home.

Anne's entire course of treatment took about a year, and I'm pleased to say that it was a success. She hasn't had a panic attack since our treatment was complete. She is able to sleep between seven to nine hours every night. Her self-esteem is much higher. She reports being much more productive at work and not overwhelmed and exhausted at the end of every day. She has a stable relationship with her husband, and he is relieved that she is not so hard on herself anymore. She does not go into fight-or-flight mode in response to an interpersonal problem. Anne's life is significantly better, and that's great. What gnaws at me, though, is the delta between what is and what could have been.

I first saw Anne as a patient when she was 45, more than 40 years after her initial ACE. If someone with her history had come to me today as a five-year-old just in placed into foster care, that child would probably have only needed three months of treatment, and a fraction of the work, and they wouldn't have grown up as Anne did, with low self-esteem and self-efficacy issues.

With that very different childhood, maybe it wouldn't have taken Anne seven years to complete her undergraduate degree, and she might have pursued an advanced degree. Her entire physical and behavioral development might have followed a different course. For instance, we could have prevented or treated other health issues like obesity that she struggled with her whole life. If she had treatment earlier, Anne would have had a much easier life, without the stress-triggered physical inflammation and all its heavy, long-term burdens on her mind and body. It's also true that while we were able to rebuild Anne's brain, later in life her health may still be compromised because she spent so much time in an inflammatory, stressed out state during her development.

The lag-time between ACEs and initial treatment is very important. The longer the lag, the greater the work required, and the longer it takes to undo the damage. Because of the nature of ACEs, the sooner the better. And thankfully, because of education and awareness, people who are suffering as a result of the effects of ACEs are coming for help sooner now.

Evolution

There was a movie a while back called *Idiocracy*. The plot was that stupid people were breeding rapidly, while smart, educated people waited too long and missed the window to have children. In the movie, the result was that the world was getting dumber and dumber.

In reality, that's not happening, thankfully. Researchers have found evidence that the average adult is significantly smarter today than they were fifty years ago.[24] Humans have an innate drive to improve, create, innovate, and evolve, and this is good news as we redefine how we understand and treat our stress.

It's a part of our human evolution to address and *solve* the stress problem. We can begin by reducing the allostatic overload that accumulates for traumatized high-ACEs children as they are exposed to chronic stress, so their brains can develop in a healthy way, instead of becoming hyper-vigilant and reactive. If we can do this, if we can swoop in and solve stress right at the moment when that first drop of mercury hits the pond, we'll be improving the evolution of the human condition. The stress problem is the root of most of our problems as a human race. If we can correct that, then we're in business.

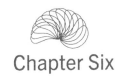

Chapter Six

NO RHYME, EVEN LESS REASON

Your nervous system is elegantly designed, but it's dumb. It's like artificial intelligence. It learns from inputs and outputs, and then does what it's designed to do. It's constantly adjusting to new information, and to hack into that, you can simply change its algorithm and direct it in a different way.

Avoidance

Another way that excess stress rears its unpleasant head is through avoidance behaviors, and there is no rhyme, and even less reason for these. At any given moment, you are unconsciously moving toward certain situations and behaviors and away from others. Avoidance begins in our fear and memory networks.

Why do we have memory as a human being? The answer begins with recognizing that everything in our body is somehow biologically adapted for the survival of our species. The purpose of memory is learning, so that we don't keep making mistakes that threaten our survival, given that our overall purpose as biological beings is to not die for as long as possible.

Fear is also necessary for survival, and is activated not only in moments when our lives are in danger, when we need to go into fight-or-flight to survive. Our fear network is also integrated with our memory network so they can work together to help us avoid stress in the future.

If I'm hiking somewhere and I start to slip next to a steep drop-off because there's loose gravel, my stress switch will trigger fight-or-flight and cement the memory of that location, the loose gravel, and drop-off for the next time I hike there. When that happens, I won't be thinking this consciously. It will be automatic, not conscious, because I went into fight-or-flight the first time and had an emotional reaction that cemented the memory. That sort of dramatic, emotional event gets embedded in my memory network differently than everyday memories. This is why you know where you were during 9/11, but you have no idea where you were the day before—unless that day was also emotionally charged.

This is also why people say to me, "I think I have a memory problem. I can't remember my childhood."

I'll ask, "Was your childhood pretty good?"

Usually, I hear, "Yes it was."

That's why they can't remember. If an incident was not emotionally charged and your stress switch wasn't triggered, you're probably not going to remember it unless somebody reminds you with a photo or story.

This is how memory works. Memory would be incredibly inefficient if you remembered every little detail of your life. Thankfully, our brain is an amazing filter. It's an amazing learner. It's an amazing integrator. This is very important with regard to the concept of avoidance. You don't have to consciously think of everything you're avoiding or moving towards because that would take too much energy. If your brain was constantly wrapped up thinking about every single thing you were purposefully moving toward or away from, you might smack your head into a wall you're moving towards on accident, because you didn't have enough bandwidth to notice it and move away.

Since avoidance behaviors are unconscious, when they show up unexpectedly it can be pretty funny, especially if you're an expert on the subject... like me.

I don't plan my lunches very effectively, because I have so much going on. Fortunately, I have an administrative assistant who makes it her job to keep me from starving to death. When I moved into a new office recently, without even thinking about it, I told her to always have the fridge stocked with fat-free turkey breasts, carrots, and club soda. I didn't need her to bring me any fancy takeout or anything like that, just plenty of those three items, and at all times. Sure enough, after we relocated she came into my office and said, "I stocked the fridge for you." I went in and looked at it, a whole fridge stuffed top-to-bottom with nothing but turkey, carrots, and club soda and thought, "This is so weird. This is weird behavior."

Then it hit me. When I was a teenager petrified of gaining weight, I would eat nothing but turkey sandwiches, carrots, and Diet Coke (which I've since swapped out for club soda). These were the only three foods I trusted to avoid gaining weight.

Now, as this is happened we were headed into summer, I had upcoming media appearances coming up that motivate me to look good, and all of a sudden I was eating like a weight-obsessed teenager again.

If I went back and processed with therapy some of the pain that I went through as the only overweight child I knew at age eight, then a teenager with body image issues, yo-yo dieting, and a crappy metabolism, in all likelihood I would start eating different things for lunch. But here I am all these years later, sticking to my dietary comfort zone because I'm still locked into the association between eating, weight, and how I look; things teenage girls are obsessed with.

This behavior was very much unconscious until the moment I opened the fridge and found it hilarious. And this is just one example.

Most of us have hundreds or thousands of little behaviors that we have no idea we do every day, or why.

The reason we avoid or move toward certain things lies in our stress switches and in our fear and memory networks, all of which record perceived threats, such as being ridiculed or gaining weight, and motivate us to act accordingly. I'm unconsciously avoiding normal lunch behavior, which is a pretty innocent pattern in terms of not having major consequences because I eat enough healthy foods; however this same pattern can create behaviors with serious implications. Moving away from healthy relationships, narrowing your life choices down because of phobias, or engaging in addictive or self-destructive behaviors to avoid emotional distress are all signs that our stress and fear has taken hold.

Not all of our avoidance patterns are unconscious. Have you ever mentioned one particular type of alcohol to somebody who once got really sick after drinking it? What was their reaction when you brought it up? They probably wrinkled their nose, or groaned at the memory of a very unpleasant night. Not only have they probably avoided that kind of alcohol ever since that incident, but they might have a physical reaction to it when you merely bring it up in conversation. If I mention Jägermeister to my best friend Katie from college, she'll make a face like she's about to be sick and let out an, "Ugh!" I know for a fact that you couldn't pay her enough to drink another shot of Jägermeister in her lifetime.

This demonstrates how powerful your avoidance system is. Nobody *needs* to drink Jägermeister, by the way. I don't even recommend it. But people do need to leave the house, drive in traffic, study for an exam, speak publicly, fly in airplanes, be around insects, apologize after they've done something wrong, and be generally functional in their lives. It's fine when avoidance patterns get locked into things that are not extremely important, like avoiding Jägermeister. But for many people, avoidance behaviors cause a lot of stress and anxiety, and they can ruin lives.

I have a patient whose sisters are very successful. He is just as intelligent as his sisters, but he is forty years old, living at home, and unemployed. The reason is an extreme avoidance pattern that includes the grocery store, public places, major streets, his own street and driveway, his front yard, and finally, anything on the other side of his front door. His stress and anxiety are so severe that they lock onto one stimulus after another, like a tractor beam in a Star Trek episode: "AVOID!" His body sends a loud and clear message about each one of those stimuli: "This is uncomfortable, so let's avoid it because it might not be good for our survival." His stress switch can go off anytime, so he sits inside his parents' house to avoid potential panic.

He had narrowed his world down so much that in the beginning of our treatment, the idea of leaving the house caused such panic that we conducted his appointments remotely, via a tele-health system. He has progressed, and we've focused on lowering his stress switch's sensitivity to leaving the house as well as the other avoidance behaviors he has accumulated over time. Once we can train his nervous system to stop signaling avoidance by setting off fight-or-flight symptoms like racing heart, sweating, and panic, his salience network will be able to restore itself to normal functioning, and he will be able to go about his life without panic.

Now let's say some well-meaning person were to come over and try to force this man to leave the house before he's ready. That would probably not end well. In those cases, the surge of stress chemicals and hormones can actually hit such highs that the person's vital signs skyrocket and they can go into shock. This is an old method called "flooding" that psychologists used to try; but we know better now: exposure to an extreme stressor without lowering the stress response during that time can seriously backfire.

Fish provide great examples of this stress overload because they have an incredibly unstable nervous system. If a fish is in its normal environment but it gets stressed out, it can experience an overload of catecholamine and corticosteroid hormones and muscle exhaustion. This is why if you take that shock to the next level by transporting them into entirely different water in a new environment, they can die. These are the same hormones that get released in our bodies when our stress switches are turned on high. This kind of stress response can kill a fish instantly. Fortunately, we're a little bit more hardy creatures than fish—it likely won't kill us immediately, but it can kill us slowly.

Avoidance Pattern Misunderstandings

In addition to the misinformed idea that you can shock a person out of their avoidance behavior and back to rational thinking, here are a few other misunderstandings I've identified around avoidance patterns.

First, it's not necessarily true that avoidance results only from traumatic negative experiences. Avoidance behaviors and even phobias can develop out of a simple nervous system reaction. Bugs are a common phobia, and where I live in Arizona we have a lot of bees. Something buzzing around can send someone into a state of fight-or-flight very quickly. (This is why I eased my children towards the giant honeycomb attached to our house rather than risking them being surprised by it). For people predisposed to phobias because of existing anxiety, the simple sound of a buzzing insect can set off a full-blown panic attack.

Cayden

Cayden, an adorable eight-year-old, entered my center with a pattern of avoiding certain activities: swim parties with friends, vacations anywhere warm, field trips to a botanical garden, and other outdoor places. Each time, he would suddenly develop a severe stomachache and be unable to leave the house. During our intake interview I discovered he was terrified at the possibility of insects showing up anywhere outdoors; he had developed an avoidance pattern around any potential situations where that could happen. His parents went to great lengths to accommodate it, and it was all but ruining their family life.

Fortunately, EMDR therapy works quickly in children, so in four sessions we were able to reverse this pattern completely and essentially fix the problem. Now Cayden enjoys both indoor and outdoor activities and isn't suffering from the pain of severe stomachaches. Better yet, we were able to avoid costly and traumatic medical tests to try to uncover a medical cause for the physical symptoms.

Whenever there's an avoidance pattern around something that most people in life could do and enjoy, it is wise to ask, "Is this an avoidance pattern based on fear? Does it really need to be there?" Avoidance will not cure anything. It reduces the ability to overcome the anxiety, because you don't get any exposure with response prevention. But you don't have to expose yourself to the feared situation to make the fear go away.

There are a few ways to overcome mild avoidance behaviors without therapy. Children often can't distinguish excitement from fear, so a parent or adult can create what I call a motivational exchange. Let's say a child is initially motivated to avoid something, like roller coasters, because his stress switch is activated when he's standing at the bottom, looking up wide-eyed at the towering drops and giant loops, listening to people screaming at the tops of their lungs. If you can create a tempting award for the child to anticipate as part of the experience, this will involve the pleasure center, and his mind can associate the fear with excitement. He may just get on that roller coaster.

You might be asking, "Who cares if a child goes on a roller coaster or not?" and you would be right, if the child's fear and avoidance began and ended right there at the amusement park. But even in the short term, simply experiencing the unchecked fear of the roller coaster might have partly spoiled an otherwise fun day at the amusement park. By finding a way through the fear and preventing the avoidance behavior, he is developing a tool he can use in other situations. Ultimately, by addressing the fear rather than giving in and avoiding the roller coaster, the child will set down an overall life path of less fear and more joy than if he had settled into a pattern of avoiding anything that caused anxiety.

When you're going to great lengths to avoid things, notice that there's a block and look at it. Sometimes avoidance is just good common sense. If I'm on that hike I mentioned and I step on loose gravel and there's a big drop off, maybe I don't want to hike in that particular area again because it may be unsafe. But if I don't notice that context and take a close look at it, my brain might misunderstand the fear it records as a fear of hiking, not a fear of dangerous drop-offs, and then I might find myself in the future avoiding *all* hikes. My brain could end up creating a generalized pattern of avoiding hiking, and in extreme cases, all outdoor activities. This is essentially what happens in the development of phobias.

The second avoidance pattern misunderstanding occurs when people react to and avoid specific bad things that they could *imagine* happening, even if nothing bad has actually happened. Remember, in these situations, it's not helpful to play the "should" game and tell the person that their fear makes no logical sense. If their nervous system has locked its tractor beam on a fear, whether real or imaginary, the fight-or-flight reaction that it kicks off in their body is one hundred percent real. When someone imagines something, their nervous system reacts the exact same way that it would if that thing were actually happening in real life. The nervous system does not differentiate between real or imagined threats.

Jealousy is a really good example of this. When a patient tells me she's having a hard time with the almost-overwhelming jealousy she's feeling toward her partner, I begin by asking if her partner ever betrayed her trust. If the answer is yes, that's a clear trauma we would treat in a specific way. But if she says no, then we look at what fear inside her is driving that jealousy. She may be afraid that her partner might cheat, or might end the relationship, or something else that would be unbearable to think about. That fear can just as powerful as if her partner actually *had* done something, because her fear system is involved. We still have to deal with that. The bottom line is that the fear exists in her body and her body is reacting the only way it knows how—rhyme or reason be damned.

The third avoidance pattern misunderstanding involves overgeneralization and children. Children are not little adults. A child's stress mechanism is more prone to overgeneralizing and avoidance patterns if they feel any level of nervous reactivity. So, if one man has been cruel and abusive to a child, all men could evoke a fight-or-flight response. The adult brain is better at discriminating between things based on context and nuances, but children don't have the categorical abilities to be so nuanced.

Let's say I'm an adult walking late at night in a dark alley in New York City, and a shady-looking character jumps out of the shadows, yells at me, and I smell alcohol on his breath. A fear response might be reasonable in that situation. But that fear won't activate my stress switch the following week when I'm walking in a suburban alley during the day, because I'll have compartmentalized that one incident and put it into context—dark alley, drunk person, big city. My daytime walk in the suburbs doesn't fit that description, so my adult brain and nervous system will discern the difference and my stress switch will remain off.

A child's brain can't calculate such nuances, so when they go through trauma, their brains will overgeneralize their fear response. Children with overgeneralized avoidance patterns from unprocessed traumatic experiences and ACEs are prone to anxiety, sleep disorders, digestive problems, and behavior issues stemming from the stress switch being on too much. And if we can't even teach adults to manage their behavior while in fight-or-flight, good luck expecting children to manage theirs.

Most people don't realize that the things they choose to move toward or avoid are very much determined by that fight-or-flight mode, that nervous system reactivity. Even once we do recognize the involuntary responses at work, it requires a process to override it— since, as we know, we can't simply outwit it.

Here's another example of fight-or-flight fear causing unconscious avoidance of imagined bad outcomes. My nephew is a high school sophomore and is such a talented baseball player that a recruiter from Stanford came out to watch him play. My nephew was excited until he looked at the requirements at Stanford, and found out they require extra foreign language credits compared with other schools. Well, he previously had such a bad experience with a Spanish teacher that he was ready to write Stanford off, giving in to his avoidance urge to put as much space between himself and Spanish class as humanly possible. While he told me about the situation, I placed TouchPoints in his hands. As he continued, his stress started to lessen—along with the impulse to avoid Spanish. Once his stress switch was firmly in the off position, he realized spontaneously how illogical he had been, and saw what a big opportunity he'd almost given up! "Why wouldn't I try for Stanford?" He suddenly asked. "I can pass Spanish, easy." He handed the TouchPoints back, completely unaware of how they might have produced the change in his thinking.

The stories and examples of avoidance patterns leading to illogical decisions, with no rhyme and even less reason, are endless. Fear of flying always seems to make it to the top of people's lists. As I'm writing this, a woman was recently killed on a Southwest flight when a piece of shrapnel went through the window, leading to a loss of air pressure in the cabin, and partially pulled her out the window. It was an awful tragedy. But now I'm seeing stories of people altering their plans because of this one isolated incident. Some are cancelling flights while others are refusing to sit in window seats.

You've probably seen the statistics showing how much more likely it is to get killed in a car accident than on an airplane, and while I'm not aware of the research regarding airplane deaths in window versus aisle seats, I'm sure it's not based on one incident. After isolated tragedies like this, people overestimate risk in similar situations and avoidance patterns set in. This was a tragic accident, and my heart goes out the family that lost their wife and mother. And it's also unfortunate that people's fear networks create unnecessary avoidance based on a miniscule probability of something happening in the future. The threat is so small that it doesn't warrant doing anything different at all, and the appearance of avoidance behavior in the face of such unlikely odds really demonstrates how the fight-or-flight fear response can go haywire.

Threats that do warrant behavior changes include things like texting while driving, eating poorly, living a sedentary lifestyle, and smoking cigarettes. So if you're supersizing your order in the fast food drive-thru while you're also on your phone changing your upcoming airline seat assignment from window to aisle—that's a perfect of example of your fear network triggering avoidance patterns based on no rhyme and even less reason.

What you avoid or move towards isn't always logical. Your fear system defies logic, and that's the whole point of it. Logic requires too much mental energy. Our fear network is doing its job perfectly, managing all of this for us without requiring logic, completely based on our body's ability to sense and react to information.

We can't take the fear response out of the equation. If we could, we'd all be logical and rational, all the time. Our elegantly designed nervous systems are unfortunately also dumb. And the flip side of avoidance is also why anything can become a behavioral addiction:

moving toward things that aren't necessarily good for us, with no rational reason. There's a reason, but it's irrational. And we often *don't* avoid things that we *should,* based on our nervous system reactivity to that particular situation, or in that particular moment. We don't avoid over-eating, we don't avoid texting while we're driving, and so on. Very few people buy cars that have the highest safety rating based on those criteria alone. Some of us do look at *Consumer Reports.* But then at the end of the day, we make a lot of judgments based on how we feel in the moment. Just ask my convertible!

I can almost guarantee you that at least one person cancelled their airline flight after hearing about the Southwest incident, decided to rent a car instead, and picked out a flashy model that wasn't very safe but looked really hot flying down a highway. Then, as they drove out of the rental car lot, they pulled out their phone and started texting as they merged into speeding traffic. The good and bad news is,that's not all their fault. Their nervous system, like their choice of vehicle, is custom-made to be irrational.

The Myth of Rational

Bitcoin is currently the big exciting thing *du jour.* Some people think it's a scam, while others think it's the early days of Apple stock, the stuff of time machine fantasies ("if only I knew then what I know now...") The excitement of possibility and the fear of missing out activates our collective stress switches, which partially explains why bubbles exist in marketplaces. When we get fearful and excited, each one of us loses reason, and a united state of irrationality begins.

We do know that people make better decisions, including stock picks and financial decisions, when they're calm. We also know that there are CEOs and traders using TouchPoints while they're deciding what to do about Bitcoin. So if you want to be rational in exciting times, read on.

This is important, because there is no such thing as totally rational thinking in the presence of stress and collective hype. Interestingly, individuals with autism tend to make the most rational stock picks. Researchers think one reason why is their emotional responses do not influence their decision-making in the same way they do for people who are not on the autism spectrum.[25] So, if you want somebody who can execute stock trades with more predictable results, you could look to people who are autistic. They don't get caught up in stock market hype and emotion and make decisions like, "Oh, this company is so exciting! I should cash out my 401K and invest in it," without doing the research. They don't get caught up in all these irrational feelings, because they feel differently and make decisions differently. And that has everything to do with the salience network.

When things have high risk and potential high reward, people make irrational decisions. The potential for high reward creates feelings of excitement, while the high risk ensures that their stress switch is now involved. Irrational thinking is partially modulated by how much nervous system reactivity is going on in the moment.

When your stress switch is off, you are totally calm, present and focused. This is when you are most rational, and capable of making your best decisions. Then, when you start to worry about something, your stress switch begins to activate. Your mind starts to conjure up thoughts, your salience network processes needs and kicks out body sensations, and your stress switch cranks up higher and higher. As it does, your level of rational thinking gets proportionally lower; the more you're stressed, the less clearly you're thinking. The better you learn to accurately assess whether your stress switch is off or on— and on to what degree—the better-equipped you'll be to know when you're not in the best position to make good decisions.

Let me illustrate this at my own expense. It was the second night after I'd moved to a foreign country, and the fire alarm went off in the house at 2 A.M. Completely disoriented, I leapt out of bed and ran down the stairs. A few steps down, apparently my legs forgot how to operate correctly, and I tumbled the rest of the way down, spraining my ankle. Fight-or-flight mode and coordination don't work well together.

Later on, some trying-to-be-helpful person said, with perfect logic, "Well, your children were upstairs; why did you run downstairs?"

Now, I'm sitting there trying to play back in my mind an incident that, let's be honest, was a live wire (me) surfing down a slippery staircase of adrenaline.

I fumbled. "Well, yes, I guess I was thinking I could turn the alarm off, because the alarm was downstairs. Or maybe that everybody was already out of the house, and I was the last to wake up."

This was a complete lie of course, because the truth was, I wasn't thinking AT ALL! My thinking brain was totally shut off. I was in survival mode, and my body was trying to keep me alive. My body ran downstairs without my brain, which was still sleeping in bed. I was a train with no conductor, barreling down the tracks. Nobody home.

Of course I was not rational, and there was no way I was going to remember what I was thinking. A brain in full-blown stress switch reactivity mode meant I wasn't thinking at all. Our bodies are specifically adapted this way as a result of the conditions that our species has faced for most of its existence; who has time to be doing pros-and-cons lists and flowchart projections when they're being chased down a hill by a river of molten lava?

Here is another example that highlights how the stress switch can disconnect rational remembering: a crime scene witness who is asked to describe the suspect and sequence of events. On a neuroscience panel, I was once asked, "Dr. Serin, when you're trying to get people to recall these things after a crime or whatever, what's the best method?"

My answer was, "Get them as calm as possible before you ask questions."

Why? Your brain shuts off anything nonessential when your stress switch is on so it can do what it needs to do. A witness to a crime was, first of all, likely in fight-or-flight mode during the crime. The encoding of events during stressful times is less accurate—what is more important: taking good notes, or getting out alive? Furthermore, when you ask them to recall the incident, they will return to a stressed state, which will make recalling any details they did record more difficult. Therefore, when attempting to get any semblance of accurate data from a witness, your best bet is to get them calm, at which point they may be able recall details tucked deep in their memory network that they would otherwise not have access to. Remember, it's not necessarily that your brain didn't record the details of what happened around you, it's that your salience network is blocking them out of your conscious thought in favor of more important concerns.

One notable exception to the rule about fight-or-flight shutting down the rational, thinking brain is when someone is specifically and extensively trained to perform effectively in high-stress situations. Soldiers and first responders, for instance, receive intense and consistent training and practice so that when they are in situations that set off an average person's stress switch, they can still perform. Think of how skillfully and calmly Captain "Sully" Sullenberger was able to perform under the most stressful circumstances when he landed his failing aircraft on the surface of the Hudson River in 2009. With both engines out, he performed a near-perfect water landing in a jet aircraft designed to land on dry tarmac, and without a single life lost. My guess is that his ability to effectively perform under such extreme pressure was the result of intense tactical practice for unplanned situations gained during his training as an elite military fighter pilot and his many thousands of hours in the cockpit. And let's not forget—some people have amazing skills and abilities, and the world is a better place with them in it.

Pleasure Principle

Your mind and body are always connected, but when you are calm, you have access to higher-order thinking, which makes you more logical. When you are stressed, lower-level brain networks take over, and signals from your pleasure centers are more likely to get carried out into action—and they can hijack rational thoughts, too. This is another reason why people do things they know are bad for them. Why? Because it feels good in the moment, and the consequences seem abstract and distant at the time. When the stress switch is on, the lizard brain is in charge, and the lizard brain makes choices based on safety, pleasure, and reward. To the people around them, however, their pleasure principle-driven behavior is completely misunderstood.

They'll say, "I just don't understand. He keeps drinking alcohol. Even though knows he's going to lose everything." Yes, because in the moment that he reaches for a drink, the brain networks in control aren't operating on rational thought.

This is a reason why habits are so hard to break. In the same way that negative experiences signal unconscious avoidance, whatever has been pleasurable in the past signals for you to do it again! And if you're stressed, rational thought goes by the wayside, to boot. Then, you have a double whammy: signals from your pleasure centers tell you to DRINK! EAT! SPEND! GAMBLE! Meanwhile there's no thinking brain on duty to put the brakes on and insert rational thought.

This also helps explain why people with ADHD are more prone to addiction. Their impulse control mechanisms and reward pathways are wired differently. It's kind of like having Tesla acceleration and

Yugo brakes. There's an internal mismatch in brain function that creates impulsivity, while their reward network responds differently in a way that makes it harder to stop certain things. When they drink alcohol, use drugs, or even steal, there's a rush of excitement at first. The thrill and the resulting feelings get embedded in the memory networks, and they're likely to repeat the behavior again without considering the consequences. And it's not that they don't know the consequences, it's just that in the moment, making the logical behavioral choice isn't a match for the more powerful networks in charge of pleasure seeking and rewards. "Yup," I had one friend say while taking a drag of a cigarette, "This is probably going to kill me someday."

This is also true of teenagers because the part of the brain that processes consequences isn't fully developed until around age twenty-five. Teenagers will take more risks and engage in adrenaline-seeking behaviors, get the pleasure that comes from those behaviors locked into their nervous system, repeat them, and get into trouble. This pattern is more pronounced with boys than girls because of differences in brain and biology that dictate behavior.

And here's the kicker: no matter what their age, no matter if someone has ADHD or not, it's the stress switch that determines whether or not the pleasure center will win over the thinking brain. The amount of stress you're experiencing alters the power of these networks and dictates cravings, impulses, and whether or not someone is likely to think before they act.

Gary

Gary, a fifty-eight year-old recovering alcoholic, had been sober for thirty years and was doing well professionally and financially. He had a great family and a lot of friends. But when his mother died, stress sent him right back into a tailspin of drinking.

Why is this pattern so common? When you are stressed, you crave regulation in the form of relief. And since most of us don't understand that the stress switch works like a dimmer, with calm at one end and panic at the other, our brains send impulses for us to get relief in ways we've felt relief before. For an alcoholic, it's alcohol. For a compulsive gambler, it's gambling. For someone with obsessive-compulsive disorder, it's repeating or checking something until the stress goes away temporarily. This pattern is true for any behavior. If you're thirsty and you don't get a drink of water, your brain will keep signaling the impulse to drink water. If you don't drink something, it will eventually become so strong that you will not be able to focus on anything else. Your body is designed to initiate behaviors necessary for survival. But if you are stressed out, your body wants to regulate that too. Believe it or not, as much as we've been talking about the sensitive salience network and how it seems to take joy in tripping your internal fire alarm, your body actually *wants* to bring you back a state of calm. To do that, it goes into your memory network and asks, "What has calmed you down before?" Enter the addiction cycle.

Alcohol, drugs, and other self-destructive behaviors can be calming. I treat a lot of people with social anxiety, and I've noticed that many of them have developed alcoholism. Alcohol was the thing that relieved the stress of being in a social environment for them. That feeling was so powerful that it got locked into their nervous system as an addiction. The addiction was created by their brain as a way of regulating their stress, and became a powerful reward.

Attempts to regulate stress are capable of creating these pleasure-driven addictions. When somebody is dealing with an addictive pleasure *and* they're stressed out, they have something to regulate and they're not thinking clearly.

My team and I were at the gigantic Consumer Electronics Show (CES) and the TV show *Shark Tank* was also there, casting for future shows. The casting director was extremely stressed out, and she heard about us and about our TouchPoints devices. She came to us and asked to try them, and of course, got relief almost immediately. Then I noticed her colleague, a petite little thing, standing there with a huge donut—the size of three regular donuts.

I looked at the donut, and then at her, and said, "Are you going to eat that?"

She nodded hesitantly, frowning. I could see the stress on her face. She pointed to the set of TouchPoints I was holding and said, "I want to try those. I'm really stressed out." I placed them on her wrists. A minute later I could tell she was feeling better, she was smiling and we were chatting up a storm.

I said, "You don't want to really eat that donut, do you?"

She looked down as if just noticing she was still holding it, "Oh my gosh, I just thought that! I don't want to eat this donut! This is disgusting. What is this? This is like a thousand calories. What was I thinking?"

I said, "You weren't thinking. You were trying to regulate your stress. I know you don't eat like this normally because you're about a hundred pounds soaking wet, and you look really healthy."

She agreed, "No, I don't. This is such a stressful week for us because we have to tell people whether or not they can get on the show."

She looked down at the donut again and back up at me.

"Yeah—I must have been out of my mind. I totally don't want it."

And with that, the donut went in the trash.

It wasn't entirely her fault, remember. Her stress sent an error message to her brain, telling her something that wasn't true—that she needed to eat what was possibly the largest donut I've ever seen. (Homer Simpson's head would have exploded in bliss!)

Switch Your Energy

No matter how avoidance or regulation patterns are playing out in your life, whether it's a fear of bees, procrastination, chasing pleasure, full-blown addiction, or crippling phobias, once you tone down your nervous system reactivity by removing excess stress, you can open up a whole new world. Imagine a life where you're not constantly being pulled toward or away from situations for irrational reasons beyond your control.

I've seen this happen with TouchPoints, neurofeedback, and the other therapies I've mentioned. I've seen people go from living in an anxiety-ridden, closed-off world to removing their stress and being whole people again (or sometimes for the first time in their lives). I've seen phobias, fears, and avoidance progress and spiral somebody's life down into a narrow prison, and then seen them spiral all the way back up and get their life back on track using these methods.

Nikola Tesla said, "If you want to find the secrets of the universe, think in terms of energy, frequency, and vibration." That's what I believe TouchPoints can do. Change the frequency, vibration, and the energetic balance and allocation within the brain and the body. When TouchPoints turn the stress switch off, that shifts the body's energy internally and externally. That energy shift is a hack to override our natural but completely irrational nervous system response. TouchPoints might just be our best shot at taking control of our elegantly designed—but *really* dumb—nervous system, anytime and anywhere.

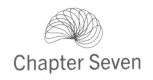

Chapter Seven

COGNITIVE DISTORTIONS

"Cognitive distortions are simply ways that our mind convinces us of something that isn't really true."
–John M. Grohol, PsyD

We all want to believe we are rational, objective people, and that we make decisions based on logical information or intuitive feelings that must be correct. However, this is not the case! Cognitive distortions, simply put, are beliefs that we think are accurate but simply aren't.[26] They fuel anger, frustration, negativity, and rigid thinking. And when you're stressed, guess what? Those distortions are more likely to take hold. That's why they are important to cover in our discussion of stress.

Here's a rundown of some common cognitive distortions that can be caused by or perpetuate the cycle of stress. As you read them, it's helpful to think about the situations in your life where these cognitive distortions might be turning up your stress switch.

#1: Filtering

Filtering happens when you magnify negative details while filtering out the positive aspects of situations. That's what my office administrator was doing when she was looking at postoperative photos of people with skin cancer right after she was diagnosed. She was filtering out the likely positive outcome of having no scars a month after surgery and staying focused on the negative of what her face would look like immediately after.

Her stress switch was on, and her thinking brain was off, so her brain filtered out the positive in favor of the negative. She wasn't doing it on purpose, and no amount of reasoning from me would have made it through to her conscious brain—she would not have heard me. When you're in a stressed state, reasonable arguments sound like Charlie Brown's teacher in the Peanuts cartoons—a meaningless "muah muah muah muah" muted trombone sound. I could have given her facts about her surgery until I was blue in the face, but it would not have mattered a bit. Cognitive distortion would have blocked out every single word.

Fortunately, for her, we had TouchPoints! Once her stress was lessened by holding a pair of TouchPoints, her conscious brain re-emerged from hiding, her cognitive filter deactivated, and she was able to process the positive photos, and feel better about the reality of her situation. With the devices in her hand, her stress switch turned off, and she could recognize the facts: she had a great doctor, eventually her healed scars would be invisible with makeup, and early detection meant no long-term threat to her life. And that's what happened. Without TouchPoints to reduce her stress, she would have suffered with undue fear in the meantime.

#2: Polarized Thinking

Polarized thinking is also called black-and-white thinking. Your brain distorts your point of view to make you believe that there is no middle ground, and sorts all of your thoughts into either/or categories, such as good/bad, easy/impossible, always/never, or love/hate. Polarized thinking is a particularly harmful form of negative thinking, and—surprise!—it amplifies even more when someone is stressed out.

You can sometimes spot this distortion by the polarizing category words, like "always" and "never." My nine-year-old son Connor was mildly upset the other day, telling me, "Mom, you *never* give me soda, *ever!*" I pointed out that he gets soda on special occasions and during some events and listed several times he recently drank soda. But I wasn't upset at the false accusation—I recognized that it's a common distortion that even adults make when they are upset.

This type of "always and never-ing" surfaces a lot when couples are in therapy. It's the all-or-nothing thinking that fuels resentment. However, when you de-activate your stress switch, suddenly the black-and-white thinking fades to shades of gray, and your thinking brain is able to see options beyond all-or-nothing.

Cognitive distortions can occur automatically, and are especially prevalent when the stress switch is on. You can't undo them or will yourself to think clearly and logically. Remember, the logical part of your brain is shut down when you're stressed (recall my tumble down the stairs in the middle of the night).

A traditional therapist might have asked my office administrator, "Do you notice that you're doing some filtering there, and you're thinking is very negative because you're only looking at the photos of people right after surgery? Why don't you consider the other photos, of people further post-op without scars, then take a few deep breaths and tell me how you feel?"

My assistant might have been able to do that; but probably not, since her stress switch was on and her lizard brain was lost in the distortion of all-or-nothing, polarized thinking.

You cannot consciously shift thoughts very well when stressed. We've been looking at it backwards, trying to shift our thoughts in the hopes of reducing stress, when the answer is to reduce stress so we *can* shift our thoughts. And in many cases once we are calm, our thoughts shift spontaneously. **My solution is this: let's lower the stress response first, and then try to shift the thought.**

#3: Overgeneralization

Overgeneralization happens when someone comes to a general conclusion based on a single incident or single piece of evidence. Just because something happened once, we shouldn't necessarily expect it to happen over and over again; but this cognitive distortion will cause someone to conclude just that.

Remember my nephew who didn't want to take another Spanish class, even if it meant missing out on the opportunity to go to Stanford? He was overgeneralizing. Because he'd had a bad experience in one class, he was afraid that he would have a bad experience in all subsequent Spanish classes. To avoid that pain, therefore, he thought he should avoid all Spanish classes. But once his stress was reduced, he was able to undo that cognitive distortion in a split second, think rationally, and make what was ultimately a better decision for his future. And this all happened automatically: once his stress was lowered, his thoughts shifted.

#4: Catastrophizing

After the Southwest Airlines tragedy where engine shrapnel went through the window and killed a woman, my friend who was going on a trip worried that the same exact situation would happen to her. In a state of stress, she was one of those who switched her window seat to an aisle. That irrational choice was an example of a *combination* of distortions (many times this is the case). First, she was overgeneralizing—if it happened once, it may happen again; or worse, it may happen to me. Second, she was catastrophizing: the absolute belief that something awful is going to happen. My friend became so stressed, and therefore so convinced that something catastrophic would happen to her if she flew in an airplane, that she nearly cancelled her trip altogether. Her stress-switched, irrational lizard brain distorted the facts into a belief that something bad was certain to happen on her flight—all based on one tragic, but extremely isolated, incident on that one Southwest flight. That is textbook catastrophizing.

People sometimes ask me how much of a gut instinct (or women's intuition, or whatever you want to call it) is actually over-reactive stress, cleverly disguised as a legitimate warning sign. That's hard to answer, because I can't choose a specific percentage. But I will remind you of the importance of tuning in and making yourself intentionally aware of whether you're in a state of stress before making any important decisions. If you tune in to your body and detect signs of stress—like increased breathing or heart rate, muscle tension, or racing thoughts—before you're hit with a hunch, there's a good possibility that it's a reaction to stress. Before you convince yourself to trust your hunch, get calm and reassess. You might find that your partner didn't text you because his phone actually was dead; you weren't invited to the party because you missed the email, rather than because your friend intentionally excluded you; or travel really is safe, even though you felt nervous about it.

One of the reasons my friend even knew about the Southwest story was because of our 24-7 easy access to the news. As human beings we are not designed for a constant stream of news. We are not hard-wired to know about every catastrophe happening that we have no control over. That's just fuel for the stress switch's fire.

People who constantly have the news on may not realize that they're bringing a lot of stress into their homes. They are flooding their nervous systems and salience networks with visual and auditory stimuli about murders, car chases, fires, and other highly stimulating pieces of information. And most of the information isn't needed for our survival—if we weren't watching the news, we would not know about all these things, and in all likelihood, our lives would not be affected—at all.

#5: Representativeness Heuristic

This is another one you might be familiar with. Heuristics are generalities that our brain uses as shortcuts so we don't have to think individually about every little thing. The representativeness heuristic is a cognitive distortion that allows you to conclude that a portion you can see is representative of a whole that you cannot.

Have you ever bought a new car and then suddenly you looked around and noticed that more cars on the road seem to be your car's make and model, even though you'd never noticed that before? This is because your salience network relies on heuristic shortcuts to decide what to notice. Before, your salience network quite efficiently filtered the make and model of nearby cars out of your consciousness to avoid using bandwidth that was needed elsewhere.

That particular car is now salient to you because it's now relevant in your life. However, if you don't recognize that this form of cognitive distortion is now in play, you might look around, see your car everywhere, and conclude that statistically speaking, more people are driving your make and model than you would've estimated before. You may even pat yourself on the back, feeling validated for your taste in choosing such a popular car.

Sorry to burst your popularity bubble, but this is all happening because your trusty salience network was filtering out specific information that it's suddenly allowing through to your consciousness. Now you see a little information you didn't see before, and conclude that reality has changed.

Representative heuristics can fuel catastrophic thinking. When you constantly watch disasters and other stressful news stories, your stress switch struggles to stay firmly in the off position. From there, it's easy to slip into overgeneralizing, catastrophizing, and overestimating the dangers of the world we live in, personalizing the stories by imagining if the bad thing happened to you, and finally fortune-telling, predicting that the story on the news will absolutely happen to you in the near future.

My advice is to pay attention to the stimuli you surround yourself with, as it has a profound impact on your functioning!

#6: Personalization

If somebody cuts me off in traffic, I don't get usually get upset. You know why I don't get upset? Because I'm sure there have been times when I've accidentally not seen somebody and cut them off. If I did, I know it was an honest mistake, because I am not an aggressive driver. I don't take things like driving, where there really is no interpersonal connection or intentional interaction, personally. However, with your stress switch in the on position, it's easy to suffer from this cognitive distortion.

I had a friend once who, whenever somebody cut him off, he would get furious and start ranting, "Stupid jerk, what does he have against me?" In a knee-jerk reaction, he would instantly take it personally, making the absolute assumption that the driver in the other car was out to get him. Sometimes he'd even pull up next to the other driver, ready to flip him or her off, only to find an elderly woman who could barely see over the steering wheel, or someone talking on their cell phone, or singing with the radio, or daydreaming in their own world. Clearly drivers like this did not cut him off intentionally as a personal insult. Realizing this would be an instant letdown for my friend, especially since his stress switch was obviously on and he was ready for a fight.

When our stress switches are on we're more likely to take things personally, and conclude that people are doing things *to* us, instead of making honest mistakes. Here's something else to remember about these cognitive distortions: chronic stress will make your lizard brain more susceptible to these fallacies in the first place, but falling victim to them will also raise your stress level. So when your stress switch is on, you're more likely to take things personally—and when you get in the habit of taking things personally, you're more likely to stay stressed.

#7: Control Fallacy

We really, really want to believe we have more control over the things happening around us than we actually do. The fallacy of control can go both ways. We can feel externally controlled, tending to see ourselves as helpless victims of fate. This can lead to a high level of stress if we believe we don't have any control over our own life.

On the flip side, an internal control fallacy makes you think you have control of things you really don't. You're assuming responsibility for the pain and happiness of everyone around you, asking, "Why are you unhappy? Is it because of something I did?" Co-dependence occurs where people overestimate their sense of responsibility for making people happy around them. This certainly leads to increased stress and eventually, burnout.

#8: Fallacy of Fairness

Another cognitive distortion that increases stress involves believing that things in life should be fair, and that when they're not, we should get upset. This distortion puts the responsibility for events in our life onto other people and allows us to pin the blame on others when things don't work out as we feel they should. The disappointment or failure activates our stress switches, and this fallacy allows us to shove the discomfort off onto another. This is another common one I see in couples' therapy!

Within our own fallacies of fairness, we each have internal rules about what others should and should not be doing. And then, when those expectations aren't met, on turns the switch and we feel perfectly justified in lashing out at others.

#9: Emotional Reasoning

Emotional reasoning occurs when we feel something and so we think it must be true. When we're stressed out, we use emotional reasoning. As in, "If I'm *this* upset about my upcoming flight, I should change my seat from window to aisle. I wouldn't be this upset if I weren't actually in danger. It must be a sign."

The next level of emotional reasoning is always trying to be right and trying to force our opinion onto others. That's also more likely to happen when our stress switches are on.

Let's say that a husband and wife need to resolve a relatively minor household issue. If the wife is already feeling stressed as a result of something unrelated that happened earlier in the day, she is more likely to take a juvenile stand with her husband, dig in her heels, and try to be right during the discussion. Her stressed out stance might be, "Damn it, my husband had better agree with me or there will be hell to pay!" But remarkably, if she weren't stressed, she might be perfectly capable of resolving the same issue without any problems at all.

Emotional reasoning can make people act like they have split personalities (as many a person in a relationship will tell you). You might say that the thinking brain takes the high road while the lizard brain takes the low road, but any time we're stressed out, we are more likely to try to prove ourselves right, and risk missing the actual issue on the table.

#10: Heaven's Reward Fallacy

The final cognitive distortion I want to cover is what is called the heaven's reward fallacy. This is where we expect our self-sacrifices to pay off, as if someone way up high above us in the sky is keeping score, and when we do good things but the rewards do not come, we feel bitter and resentful.

As with the other fallacies, there is a flip side to the reward fallacy as well. This happens when someone puts in less effort than they believe should be required to get a certain outcome, but that outcome happens anyway. Our beliefs can become distorted so that we either don't trust that the outcome is real, or we feel guilty about having something we think we did not earn. Needless to say, not trusting good things that come to us in life, or punishing ourselves for having them, will certainly ratchet our stress switches right up.

This side of the heaven's reward fallacy is interesting because it offers some insight into the problem of scientists looking at every little thing in the pond instead of the mercury that is poisoning it. We tend to think we need to complicate things and work overly hard for there to be some congruent pay off. If you believe that you have to put in X amount of work to reap Y amount of benefit, and then X turns out to be P—meaning a lot less work than you thought—it feels out of alignment for you. It feels like the reward or answer is too good to be true, given the amount of work you put in; that it should have been harder or more complicated to arrive at the solution.

The cognitive dissonance (clashing of contradictory ideas) this distorted belief creates can be very stressful for people, because it asks them to hold two conflicting thoughts in their mind: "It takes X effort to get Y reward. But hold on, it did *not* actually take X effort and

I still got Y reward anyway. This must not be real!" They'll conclude, "It was too easy. Something is off. I'm being tricked. There must be a catch."

Even scientists tend to over complicate solutions sometimes. They have been trained and programmed to believe that a complex problem like stress absolutely cannot have a simple solution.

The irony is that cognitive distortions like the heaven's reward fallacy do not occur as often in a state of calm. When you are thinking clearly, you are less likely to look for complex solutions in order to satisfy stress-triggered distortions like, "nothing good comes easy. There must be a catch."

Try telling a scientist who's been studying stress for years and years as his life's work, that he doesn't need to do that anymore, that the problem has been solved. Imagine how stressful this would be for him. In 1983, Dr. J. Robin Warren and Dr. Barry Marshall hypothesized that ulcers are the result of *Helicobacter pylori* bacteria, rather than excess acidity, and thus ulcers could be treated with antibiotics. [27],[28],[29] Turns out they were right, but it took over a decade for the medical community to accept their conclusions and turn an entire branch of medicine on its head. Can you imagine how stressed ulcer doctors had to be at that time, learning that their treatment protocols were based on erroneous thinking, and that a course of antibiotics could essentially replace their livelihood? How many, do you think, happily threw up their hands, abandoned their life's work, and admitted, "Okay, I guess we were wrong, on to solving the next thing!" And how many would you estimate stuck to the disproved theory that a combination of acid and stress caused ulcers, regardless of the new evidence, because it was the one they were committed to? Dr. Marshall even went so far as to infect himself with the bacteria and cure himself, and the medical community remained skeptical. Fast-forward to 2005, and Warren and Marshall's team received a Nobel Prize in Medicine for their work, over two decades after their initial discovery.

I understand the irony of this book. I understand how ironic it is that offering a simple solution that shifts the long-held paradigm from coping with stress to curing stress is going to *create* stress for a whole lot of people, especially treatment providers on the front lines who are going to be forced to shift their own practices and beliefs. But lucky for them, they can use TouchPoints too.

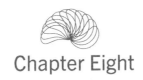

Chapter Eight

PERFORMANCE ISSUES

"A catch would have resulted in a first down. Instead, the football had bounced off his outstretched hands. 'I just didn't make the play,' Brady said."
Asked if he caught the pass in practice, he said: 'Yeah, I caught it. Didn't catch it tonight.'"
—New England Patriots Quarterback Tom Brady, after losing Super Bowl LII.[30]

When performance is high-stakes, we're more likely to go into a stressed state. Psychologists use something called the Yerkes-Dodson law to show that there is an optimal zone of arousal (stress) that produces peak performance.[31] Being a little stressed can help your performance. However once you move beyond that to an excess amount of stress, performance starts to worsen. That often looks like an athlete who "choked in the clutch."

Have you ever watched your favorite professional sports team blowing it in a championship game and thought, "Who are these people? Why does this team, who has been wiping the field with the competition all season long, suddenly look like a JV high school team chasing their tails? Have they lost their minds?"

Well, they've lost part of their minds. The make-it-or-break-it stress of a situation like the Super Bowl can set off an athlete's stress switch, robbing them of access to higher-order thinking. Even drilled-in training can fail when high-stakes situations have created a level of anxiety that all the skills and practice in the world are not able to physically override.

It's true that most of the time, an athlete's elite training and skills are able to override their nerves even when the stakes are at their highest. That's when we'll see game-winning plays, Olympic miracles, and other stories of triumph. But when we see the opposite scenario, an athlete or team choking at a clutch moment, it would be impossible to rule out the stress switch.

Think of the Olympic figure skater falling on the critical jump that would have achieved the gold medal, the golfer who nearly had the tournament wrapped up until he missed the putt on the last hole, the baseball outfielder who dropped the pop fly, or the college basketball player who misses the free throw that would have won his team the national championship game.

An athlete can make a play hundreds of times in practice and then, when the big game rolls around, inexplicably, it doesn't happen. You've probably seen press conferences where these players come to the microphone looking upset and also slightly dazed and confused; and when quizzed by reporters: "What happened today?" they stare back blankly and say, "I just don't know." I would guess these answers are total honesty; as their stress switch begins to turn off, and their conscious brain slowly firing back up again, they're honestly trying to remember what happened!

Now, most of us are not headed for the Super Bowl anytime soon. But you don't have to be an elite athlete to experience performance issues. Some ways that stress wreaks havoc on our daily performance can include taking a wrong turn and getting lost on the way to a job interview, forgetting notes at home and showing up unprepared for an important meeting, drawing a blank during a speech, or spilling red wine on yourself during Thanksgiving dinner with your new in-laws. There are countless other everyday examples of too much stress tanking performance.

In each of these situations, stress shuts down nonessential functions like critical thinking, poise, and gracefulness, so the situation can go from bad to worse. Unfortunately, your biology and DNA don't care about your job interview, meeting, speech, or dinner with your in-laws. Your biology only cares about survival, and when your stress rises, performance on these *biologically* nonessential functions goes out the window.

The level at which your brain is in fight-or-flight is directly proportional to your performance. So, if you're moderately stressed out during a test, you can remember certain things. But if you're incredibly stressed, your mind might go blank. If you're sweating bullets, and your heart is racing, you cannot think yourself back into a non-stressful state. Your brain will become unable to recall pieces of information you studied only the night before. Then, five minutes after the test ends, all the answers come flooding back into your brain! When the stress shuts off, the genius comes back.

This is where training, habituation, and practice can come into play. Rehearsing those activities conditions the brain and body to perform better in high-stress situations. People who practice more do better in high-pressure situations like the Super Bowl because their bodies recall established neural patterns in those moments. When the stress hits them like a firestorm, their bodies are more likely to perform those well-practiced motor movements.

Another way to illustrate the habituation of motor movements through practice is with driving. When you first learn how to drive, you have to think about every last detail: "Where is the brake? Are my mirrors set up? Is my key in the ignition?" Initially, you have to go through all these items one by one, which requires a lot of conscious thought. The brain networks that activate when learning something new are different than the networks that activate once something becomes habit. So once you learn to drive and your body memorizes those motor movements and sequenced patterns, there's less activation needed in your higher-order thinking brain. You don't get in your car every day and go down a driver's-ed checklist. You probably operate your car with your brain mostly on autopilot. My mom understands this phenomenon well. When she has a lot on her mind, she'll get in the car and automatically drive the route to work, only to realize, "why am I going this way? I was supposed to be going to the bank!"

Fortunately, once a task is habitual, your brain will no longer require the higher-order thinking to execute it, because it is operating in different areas of the brain. And more good news is that, just like driving, anything that is practiced enough to become automatic may be less subject to the stress override, or choke, that can happen in high-performance situations.

Working Memory

Working memory is something else that affects your performance in the moment. It refers to how much mental control you have as something is happening. Working memory is related to short-term and long-term memory, but it is not the same thing as simply recalling memories.

Simply put, short-term memory allows you to recall something that happened a few minutes ago while long-term memory allows you to recall things that happened years ago. Working memory occurs in the interval of time in which things are actually happening. So, if I say the numbers four, six, three, two, and then ask you to repeat them backwards, you would need working memory to hold the numbers in your mind while you manipulate them into two, three, six, four. Doing that requires mental control.

Your working memory is something akin to an Etch-a-Sketch in your mind, so when I gave you that list of numbers and asked you to reverse them, your mental Etch-a-Sketch was scribbling them down, first in the order I gave them to you, and then in backwards order.

How much working memory you have dictates how long you'll be able to visualize those numbers in your mind before the Etch-a-Sketch effect takes hold and they start to disappear.

Most people can remember five to nine numbers in their minds at one time. The better your working memory, the more you can remember, and the more efficiently you can learn. People with poor working memory usually have more problems learning new information, and difficulty logging it into long-term memory. Working memory underlies both of those skills, as well as overall performance. If a child has poor working memory, over time it will modulate their IQ and overall academic performance is likely to be lower in the long run.

As you might have guessed by now, there is a strong link between memory and stress. Stress modulates working memory, which means the more stressed out you are in the moment, the less working memory—and thus mental control—you have to wrangle higher brain functions. So, if working memory fluctuates according to how stressed you are in the moment, then stress, once again, is the moderating factor that determines important outcomes.

Here is another way to think about working memory and stress: picture a file cabinet in your brain that holds all your memories and learned information. Every time you want to recall a memory or a piece of information, a secretary in your brain pulls out the file, gets the information you need, and puts the file back into the file cabinet. If you're in a stressed out state, the secretary in your brain is not going to be able to access that file. When you're stressed during a test, and your mind goes blank, it's because your secretary is on strike until conditions improve.

This is key when it comes to a child's performance, because when children are stressed out while they're trying to learn, their working memory capacity is lowered. That blocks their learning in the moment, keeping them from reaching their full potential. What they're learning in that stressed out moment is likely not going to make it into their long-term memory storage, either. When the secretary is on strike, she doesn't put the files back correctly. The process of learning does not go smoothly for a stressed out child.

Stress can take a child with average working memory and intelligence and render their learning processes extremely inefficient. Stress will effectively prohibit them from harnessing their working memory and interfere with learning during the interval of time in which it should be taking place.

This would also apply to stressed out adults in learning situations at work, in trainings, classes, or even reading a book or watching a documentary on television. If you are in a state of stress, your ability to learn is impaired.

Effects of Stress on Learning

Without knowledge of the connections between memory, learning, performance, and stress, parents will insist that little Johnny has a learning disability because he is doing horribly in one school subject, let's say math. In their minds, since Johnny is doing well in all his other subjects, he must have a learning disability that is preventing him from doing well in math.

At the Serin Center clinics, the first thing we might do is to reduce Johnny's stress level, using TouchPoints and other methods, so we can see what he's capable of when he's not stressed out. In a majority of cases we've seen, the performance patterns do not replicate when we lower the stress and complete testing when a child is calm. We often find there is no actual learning disability underlying Johnny's problems in math. (Even when there is a learning disability present, lowering the stress often leads to better outcomes during interventions).

In therapy, we would find out what specifically is causing stress in math class. It might be a "mean teacher," a bullying situation, or something Johnny was told about his ability to do math. We can essentially undo the harm using bilateral stimulation with TouchPoints and EMDR therapy so Johnny does not react with stress to similar events. It's very important to do that as soon as possible after an upsetting event. I've seen children who had a mean teacher for one year in a single subject end up having problems with that subject throughout their lifespan. Memory, learning, and performance get intertwined and locked in with anxiety for life because their nervous systems memorize the message that math is a threat to survival, and therefore fight-or-flight kicks in to protect them. Remember, the elegantly designed but dumb nervous system makes no distinction between being attacked by bees and sitting in math class. Even in the future, being in a different math class with a perfectly nice teacher will kick that stress switch on, once it has been altered by a bad experience. And when the stress switch is on, learning turns off.

Outside of physical circumstances, like being in the presence of a mean teacher, anxiety can also arise from belief systems. There was a stereotype prevalent in the 1990's that girls were not as good at math as boys. It has been debunked, but the idea is still out there, and as a woman, you may have even been affected by it at some point. You might remember being told this, or maybe someone will make a joke as you're walking into a room to take a math test. No matter how this belief entered your consciousness, as a female taking a math test in an academic situation, you will probably experience stress about it and do worse on the test than you would have otherwise.

If you tell yourself (consciously or subconsciously) that you're bad at math, the idea will perpetuate and lock itself into your nervous system. Now, your cognitions and your nervous system are working in sync with each other to decrease your performance. This will continue until you uncouple your cognitions (in this case, the belief that women are bad at math) from your nervous system reaction (general stress at the thought of doing math). You might uncouple these two processes consciously, for instance through stress reduction and other therapies, or unconsciously, by finding a type of math you really enjoy.

The latter example, finding a type of math you enjoy, is an example of a motivation override. We can sometimes get over our avoidance patterns by finding a motivation that's strong enough to overpower the avoidance. Normally we try to avoid what we're afraid of, like the child avoiding the roller coaster, my nephew avoiding Spanish classes, or little Johnny avoiding math. But if we can find a motivation that's positive enough to override the fear, we're in business.

I can speak from observation that psychologists are notoriously petrified of taking statistics courses. Some of them will consider dropping out of psychology altogether because of that *one* course requirement. But most of them will power through because they're so motivated to be in the profession.

I struggled in math too, which planted the seed in my mind that I wasn't good at it. But any future performance patterns were headed off when I started studying statistics, which I loved! Statistics felt a little exciting for me because it had context and a story behind the math instead of just boring numbers that I was adding up. Once I tapped into that excitement, the motivation quickly overrode any previous anxieties about math, and the cycle of memory, learning, stress, and performance issues was broken.

Mood Congruent Memory

Mood congruent memory is the final piece of the cycle that can lead to performance issues. Memories are extremely inaccurate, because memory itself is fluid. In any given moment, when you access a memory in your mind, mood alters your perception of that memory. If it's a cloudy, rainy day and you're feeling a little down, it will be harder for you to try to remember something that happened on a sunny and bright day. How you feel about today's conditions will create an overlay onto the memory you're trying to recall. Even if the memory of the sunny day was a positive one, it'll be tainted by your current mood and conditions.

Your brain is not static. It's an integrator, meaning it brings together details from several different, similar memories, even though you think you're remembering one single memory—but you believe you're remembering it accurately. This is one way that memories are fluid and inaccurate, which is why it's so easy to implant false memories in people through the power of suggestion, hypnosis, and other means.[32] In addition, since as you've learned, your salience network chooses what to notice and what to ignore, the details your memory records may be biased. Remember that your emotionally charged memories hold more weight than ones without emotion. Stress affects what you remember, how you remember it, and how easily you're able to recall it.

The only reason I can remember my fifth birthday party is because my mom hired Chuckles the Clown. I was so excited and had all sorts of expectations of the fun my friends and I would have! Well, Chuckles turned out to be a woman who was as drunk as a skunk, with makeup smeared all over her face, and she made balloon animals that looked like intestinal diseases. My mom to this day recalls it as a funny story. I remember standing in the middle of our living room bursting into tears because this crazy woman ruined my party. Those tears, and the emotion behind them, are the reason I remember my fifth birthday party. I can, of course, chuckle about Chuckles now, but had my party been a run-of-the-mill affair, I wouldn't be able to recall it very well at all.

The secretary that files memories in your brain files memories with high emotions differently than run-of-the-mill memories. She also alters the files every time she pulls them out. Ever wonder why when someone retells a story for the tenth time, it's way different than the first version—but they swear that's exactly how it happened? Blame the secretary! When you put all this together, it's easy to see how mood has a powerful influence over what you remember and how you remember it. The phrase "your mind is playing tricks on you" takes on a whole new meaning!

The purpose of memory is not to provide you with your own perfectly accurate, crystal-clear mental Pinterest board of your life. Memory is meant to be a survival mechanism. We have to remember what to move towards and what to avoid for our survival. This is why the memory system and the fear system are good buddies. For every conscious memory, there are a multitude of unconscious ones that have been embedded in our brain, dictating what we avoid or are attracted to, and instructing our nervous system to respond accordingly.

Are you seeing why the removal of stress is so crucial to our individual performance, and bigger than that, to our full potential as human beings? In all these different ways, from slowing your thinking, to hindering your learning, to even altering your memories, stress is like mercury seeping through the day-to-day processes that influence your performance. Stress impacts mood, which shapes memory, which impacts performance, which, over the long-term, determines potential.

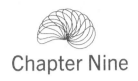

Chapter Nine

DAGGERS

"Speak when you are angry,
and you'll make the best speech you'll ever regret."
-Laurence J. Peter

Stress brings out the worst in all of us. When our stress switches are on, our thinking brain shuts off, and the consequences can run the gamut from behaviors that harm us to ones that hurt others. With words especially, a state of stress can switch off any mental filters that you think you have in place under better circumstances, and verbal daggers may fly with no thought of the later repercussions.

This is what happens when celebrities or other public figures lose it on camera, and then must issue public apologies afterwards. Even outside of instances that involved alcohol or other substances, it's easy to find examples of celebrity apologies made necessary after the individual lost control, their stress switch flipped on, and started spraying verbal daggers at people around them.

"I am happy to be the poster boy for thinking about what you say and
how those words, even if you don't intend them and how they mean, they
are rooted in hate, and that's bulls—t. I shouldn't have said that."
—Jonah Hill

"This momentary indiscretion has jeopardized the most important thing in my life."
—Kristen Stewart

"I'm sorry, as everyone who knows me is aware, for losing my temper..."
Alec Baldwin

"I was out of order beyond belief... I was way out of order. I acted like a punk."
—Christian Bale

"I had a lot of stress and you know this it's very lonely. When I think back on it, if I had to do it differently, letting people go and being mad about having to rewrite everything I was just angry a lot of the time."
—Matthew Weiner

The subtext in each of these apologies seems clear: "I don't know what happened. I don't know why I said or did these things, I must have lost control, and I regret it." The lesson anyone who has ever been in such a situation has learned is that careless daggers have serious consequences. In day-to-day life, verbal and behavioral daggers affect how we connect with others.

Turned-on stress switches lower your level of empathy and caring, disconnect you from others, and increase the chances you will hurt them with words or actions. Then, you will be mystified by your behavior after the fact, wondering what happened and how you could have done or said such things, because you know you're not a mean person. You are responsible for your behavior in general, but it's not entirely your fault. Remember that once the stress switch goes on, anything that is not critical at that moment is going to get shut off. So rational thought and impulse control give way to anger and the expression of it. Boom.

How much we are able connect with other people in a meaningful way and control ourselves in our relationships is dependent on the level of stress we're experiencing. Spending a significant amount of time in fight-or-flight can worsen relationships over time. Allowing these patterns to remain unchecked can create irreparable damage, and ultimately, put the long-term success of your relationships with your family, partner and children into jeopardy—*even if the relationship is not the main stressor.*

Having said that, however, relationships have a unique ability to trigger our stress switches. I think we've all had the experience of saying something we didn't mean in the heat of the moment, and later on, when we're calmer and feel the regret, having to apologize for our words or actions. When we are in fight-or-flight we become a different, more selfish, uncaring version of ourselves that seems unrecognizable to us when we're *not* in fight-or-flight. We become our own versions of the two-faced Dr. Jekyll and Mr. Hyde. When our stress switches are on, crazy, vindictive Mr. Hyde comes to the surface. But then, when we calm down and Dr. Jekyll reemerges, we become reasonable, regretful and apologetic. It's not that we have a split personality. It's that we have a functioning nervous system.

Parents often come to me and say, "My child is mean."

I ask, "Is she mean when she's calm?"

"No. In fact, she often blows up and then she feels very, very bad about it afterwards."

This immediately tells me that their child is not inherently mean. If a child acts mean only when her fight-or-flight system is activated, the problem is that she is being activated too often or by certain triggers.

I don't care if you are the nicest, sweetest person on the planet. You could be the next Mother Teresa, Gandhi, or Dalai Lama, but if you are a human being with a nervous system, you have the capacity to throw daggers at someone else, especially if you're in fight-or-flight. Even yogis meditating on mountaintops for eight hours a day are not immune to biology. The difference for the yogis is that their conscious decision to meditate frequently helps keep them *out* of fight-or-flight. It is their way of controlling what is mostly uncontrollable.

For some people, the inability to stay calm is a chronic, out-of-control problem. Take the dad who came in, insisting that his son had a chronic anxiety problem. We can often treat a child's anxiety beautifully. But if there's a problem in the home with one or both parents going into fight-or-flight quite a bit, the child's anxiety might return over time.

In this particular case I found out that dad was coming home every night so stressed from work that he would actively search for something to yell at the children about—if he couldn't find anything obvious like dirty dishes in the sink, or toys left out on the floor, he'd go around opening drawers and yell about them not being clean enough. His fight-or-flight system could always find something to attach to that he would explode about. The whole family, including the anxiety-ridden son, was forced to deal with those daily explosions, and of course they affected how the family functioned.

A common defense mechanism when you're around somebody who goes into fight-or flight regularly is to tell yourself, "I don't care," "This is fine," or "I'm so used to it that it really doesn't bother me anymore." Unfortunately, your beautiful, dumb nervous system is incapable of such high-level rationalizations. The stress is getting to you, whether you acknowledge it or not.

Because unless you're a sociopath or psychopath, or you have certain developmental disabilities like severe autism, you have a functioning mirror neuron network system in your brain that reflects and absorbs other people's moods. So, being in the room with someone whose stress switch is on will change *your* brain wave patterns, which in turn will affect your body's stress switch. Enduring someone else's stress this way for long enough will cause inflammation, disorders, and disease, whether or not you're being yelled at. Being around out-of-control stress is like being around someone throwing invisible daggers—even if they're not purposely aiming at you, if you're near them, you're getting hit. Stress does not exist in a vacuum. The collateral damage of stress knows no limits. *It affects everything and everyone around it.*

With this book, I am raising a red flag to elevate the conversation about stress from an individual problem to a national epidemic. Excess stress suffered by the individual is negatively impacting families, communities, groups, and our future as a society. Stress is much bigger than the self-help aisle, and it is time we treat it that way. Elevated to a national level, the daggers we throw at one another in seemingly harmless arguments could even make or break us as a nation. Entire countries can be activated to a state of reactive fear, and the daggers can be more than just heated exchanges of words. On a global level, the daggers we throw can make or break us as a species.

Anonymous Daggers

The dangers associated with verbal daggers that are triggered by stress activation are particularly heightened when word wars break out between strangers who have their stress switches on, especially on social media where nearly everyone has access and a nearly anonymous voice.

We get social media comments about TouchPoints, including snarky ones from people I can tell are not our customers and in all likelihood never will be. While I'm not going to be able to control the commenters or their comments, it is my responsibility to control my awareness of my level of stress, and therefore whether it's a bad idea for me to respond. Imagine the different responses I might have to one of those negative comments. Stress switch on: "Hey! Don't knock it 'til you try it! Did YOU spend a decade researching this and perfecting the waveform? Because I DID!" Versus stress switch off:

"Have you tried TouchPoints yet? Here's some data to look at." Taking a pause to get that switch in the off position can make a tremendous difference.

But most people aren't taking that pause, especially on social media. Log on, look at the never-ending threads beneath posts, especially political ones, and watch those daggers fly! If someone's stress switch is on and they have the instant ability to lash out impulsively, that's exactly what they will do, without giving it a second thought. There is no awareness. Social media is a breeding ground for this. If you have a thought, no matter what your mindset, you can make it known immediately.

I think this phenomenon comes down to the immediacy granted by the always-on Internet—instant access means no barriers, checks, or balances. Imagine I see something on social media that makes me very upset. But I either don't have the time or the access (maybe I've forgotten my log in) to comment on it in that moment. The likelihood that I will still have the desire to go back to that post and leave an angry comment later, when my stress switch is off, is very low.

This cocktail of content built to trigger stress (remember that our bodies are not designed to constantly absorb those negative news stories), immediate access, and the veil of anonymity can lead to outright virtual battles. There are those who log on, daggers in hand, just looking for another target whose stress switch is also on, to do battle with. Again, you can't stop *them,* as much as you'd like to try, but you can control *you.* You can tap into your new awareness of the signs that your stress switch is on—irritation, frustration, pounding heart, rapid breathing, inability to think clearly, sweating—and if it is, you can refuse to act in the heat of the moment.

This pattern of lashing out when you're stressed is the reason why psychologists advise people to save their angry emails as drafts and then revisit them later, once they're calm. In most cases this will lead to a calmer rewrite. But if you hit send while you're in an activated state, you risk sparking a battle of e-daggers flying back and forth.

These e-daggers, on social media and email, and with people we know or strangers, are big contributors to our national epidemic of stress. People seem much more willing to unleash their stress onto others in this way than to actually do something about either their stress or the issue that has activated it. As a result, stress keeps spreading, like an unseen poison.

Nuclear Daggers

Some kinds of stress-triggered daggers are more devastating than others, and some people throw daggers because they feel entitled to—which brings me to a very important point. In this discussion of "daggers," I am not talking about violence or threats in any way. The daggers I am talking about are made up of excess stress coming off another person, from a bad day or whatever is happening with them, and landing on you. If someone's stress triggers them to threaten others with verbal, emotional, or physical violence, that's not daggers, that's abuse, and it's dangerous.

Unfortunately, we can't always point to the stress switch as a cause for abuse, either. There are psychopaths and dictators throughout history who have been very calm while they inflicted pain, manipulation, and suffering on others. While *they* may not have stress to blame for their cruel actions, the stress and fear responses they cause can be catastrophic, even for those who are not direct victims.

Even outside of the cases of psychopaths and actual evil, over-reactive or impulsive daggers thrown out of fear or stress can jeopardize the security and safety of entire countries. Look at the "almost annihilation" scenarios in history, like the Bay of Pigs invasion. Years later, some leaders from the time have alluded to how, as a group, they were in a state of fight-or-flight, in fear of the threat to America, and therefore feeling they had no choice but to act from that place of fear.[33] Their thinking was prone to be antagonistic, disconnected, and non-empathetic due to the fear and stress. If the situation had escalated any further than it did, any action would have risked devastating unintended consequences, and potentially an atomic bomb. The world is fortunate that the powers-that-be calmed down, did not act in that activated state, and that the result was not annihilation.

There have been a slew of world leaders (typically not the very good ones) throughout time who have acted on important decisions out of fear and stress. Realistically, being the leader of a nation definitely falls in the high-stress job category, so it seems unavoidable that this would happen. Fortunately, outside of dictatorships, there are checks and balances to provide damage control.

For the reactive, stressed leader, though, the dangers are the same as to you and me: behavioral issues, lack of empathy, inability to connect with others, and ongoing health problems. Stress is stress, and it has the same effect on you and those around you, whether you're the dad who yells about the dirty dishes or you're ruling from a castle or the White House.

Shielding Yourself from the Daggers

What can you do to protect yourself from stress-triggered daggers thrown by others, which can in turn lead to you throwing your own? It's a good idea to identify some proactive ways to shield yourself, because otherwise your own stress switch is likely to trigger less-productive survival mechanisms like those we've already discussed. If your boss is an incredibly stressed out person, for example, you may start to avoid meetings with him, or avoid doing projects where you're going to have to work closely with him. Many oppositional behaviors start with the uncomfortable feeling of having to deal with somebody who is stressed out. That's one way that avoidance habits like procrastination and interpersonal issues at work develop. And unfortunately, because of proximity, sometimes there are stressed out people you can't simply avoid.

One year, my son Christopher had a teacher who emanated stress so strongly it was like perfume. She doused herself in it, and it affected him badly. Our children are with their teachers up to seven hours a day in a traditional public school setting, so this teacher's stress created incredible anxiety in my son. He would come home with stomachaches and not want to do school work. It would have been very easy for me to accuse him of slacking off and being lazy, and tell him to pull it together and get his work done, no matter what. I'll share with you in a bit the approach I used to solve the problem, but let's talk first about you, and what you can do in a situation like this, where avoiding the source of stress is not an easy option.

Tuning In to Your Stress Switch

Most importantly, it's a good start to practice tuning into your stress switch in various circumstances. Learn to notice the signals when it starts to flip on, and how you feel when it's off. If you know how your body feels when you're at peace versus even mildly stressed, you'll be more likely to catch yourself when your switch starts to activate. Awareness of your body's stress signals is key.

Let's say that you find yourself in the presence of a stressed out person tossing daggers, and your stress switch starts to flip on. You may notice physical signs that you are coming out of a peaceful state and going into a stressful one: perhaps your heart starts racing, your breathing speeds up, your thoughts race like NASCAR drivers, you begin to feel uncomfortable or notice yourself interrupting. As your stress switch moves upwards, you might feel pressured to say something, defend yourself, or worse, retaliate. When you become more aware of these signs, there are a few things you can do to shield yourself from the daggers and stay out of fight-or-flight.

First, as you recognize what's happening, start to take deep breaths and slow down your perception of the situation. Remember that the other person is activated, so they're speeding things up and trying to bring you with them. But that doesn't mean you have to go along for the ride and automatically play their game. You are in charge of you, so turn on your awareness, spot where you are on the stress spectrum, breathe, and slow down the scene around you. If possible, remove yourself from the situation.

If you are in danger, *definitely* remove yourself, and I will repeat a very important point—I am absolutely NOT talking about physical abuse situations here. If you are in such a situation, get out immediately and then seek help. I don't want you to mistake what I'm saying as telling you to "breathe" your way out of a dangerous situation. My aim here is to give you a strategy to shield yourself from other people who are not in control of their own stress switches, and avoid triggering yours unnecessarily.

You can learn to continuously tap into your awareness of where you are, stress-wise, when your stress switch starts to turn up, and try to consciously act to manage your own nervous system, versus reacting to someone else's. With this awareness, in theory you can choose to train your brain over time to do something different in response to stress.

Learning to notice the signs that your stress switch is being triggered comes first. You need to see the situation coming in order to try to change your response. If you can keep your stress switch from turning up too high, too fast, you may have some time to self-reflect and change your response.

However, it won't help much to see it coming if your stress switch automatically turns on too high and too fast, or if your go-to tools for change are ineffective, which has been the case with a lot of approaches. Without effective tools including EMDR, neurofeedback, and TouchPoints technology, attempting to retrain these involuntary systems takes an extreme amount of time and effort and can be downright nearly impossible.

This approach, of using effective methods alongside self-awareness to retrain the memory network's reaction to stress, is the one I ended up using in my son's situation with his anxiety-producing teacher. Talking with Christopher, I recognized the symptoms of some kind of fight-or-flight reaction and anxiety. Together, we identified that he was reacting to the teacher. Now, I wasn't in a place where I was going to have him switch schools or teachers, or other drastic, life-upending measures. What I did do though, was allow him to take a set of TouchPoints to school for a few days, so he could use bilateral stimulation to calm himself, and allow his memory to record the new experience of being around her while feeling physiologically calm.

What having both insight about his stress switch trigger and the TouchPoints did for Christopher—and this is something you can do as well— was train his nervous system to not react to stress in that specific situation. Having him intentionally calm himself—using highly effective bilateral stimulation at the level of his involuntary systems—allowed his brain to experience being calm rather than stressed in the presence of that particular stress trigger (his teacher). The TouchPoints helped him shield himself from the teacher's stress daggers by creating calm in her presence, which created a new pattern of automatic behavior, so the next time he was with her his default was calm.

That's essentially what desensitization is. Once again, an important distinction to make is that you should only do this in situations that are not personally dangerous to you. But in the case of a grumpy, stressed out teacher that my son needed to endure for the rest of the school year, the answer was to get him calm in the presence of her stress.

Immunity

Who's immune to daggers? The answer is *no one*. I have a PhD in Neuropsychology, and I'm on a Listserv with other neuropsychologists, doctors, psychiatrists, and neuroscientists where we discuss anonymous patient cases, technology, techniques, and best practices. The goal is for the group to be a private forum to talk, improve patient care, be on the cutting edge of what's going on, collaborate with professional peers, and share a better collective base of knowledge. That's the goal.

The reality? Sometimes it's more like Twitter. Yes, these are extremely smart, well-educated individuals; they must have well-developed frontal lobes and executive function control in order to have planned, organized, and executed their way through years of advanced education and clinical training to MDs and PhDs. But they're still human beings.

People with lots of letters after their names are on this Listserv fighting back and forth and insulting each other like children all the time. Respected scientists get banned from this group on a regular basis because, like the celebrities at the top of this chapter, they lose control. The same thing happens in person, and it's very, very uncomfortable. Even well educated experts in brain function have nervous systems that are run by lizard brains with stress switches firmly in the on position much of the time. I don't care how many degrees or certifications you have, you are not immune to throwing impulsive daggers when your stress switch clicks on.

I found a great case in point while attending an EMDR therapy conference several years ago. EMDR therapists are truly amazing people. They heal people daily and have made it their life's work to make the world a better place. They volunteer around the globe, working with trauma victims in third-world nations. This particular conference was packed with some really good-hearted, highly educated people.

Remember what I said about even the Dalai Lama having the biological capability of throwing stress-daggers if his nervous system was triggered? At the *very* first meeting I attended during the EMDR conference, I sat in the back of the room and watched this room full of all of my therapy heroes—really giving, compassionate people— break out in a fight! Not quite a fistfight, but the verbal daggers were pretty sharp. The heated conversation quickly turned juvenile. The level of argument wasn't very far above Twitter language. These humanitarian therapists were throwing verbal daggers akin to, "Oh yeah? I know you are, but what am I!" So next time you end up activated and catch yourself tossing daggers of your own, remember, you're in good company! Take my word for it: just because you're a sympathetic scientist doesn't mean you can't be a sympathetically activated one!

One of the smartest people in history, believe it or not, found himself unable to wrangle his own nervous system. In 1872, Charles Darwin attempted a self-study to eliminate his innate fear of snakes. He regularly went to the zoo and stared at a poisonous viper called a puff adder behind glass. Although he vowed to himself he would not move or flinch when the snake tried to strike, without fail, Darwin found himself recoiling every time the snake lunged at him even though in his conscious mind he knew it could not hurt him from behind the glass.

He noted, "As soon as the blow was struck, my resolution went for nothing, and I jumped a yard or two backwards with astonishing rapidity."

Despite using his thinking brain to try not recoil, his more powerful reptilian brain took over and he jumped back every time. Should a layer of glass not have protected Darwin, this instinct would have served him well. But even though he knew he was safe, no amount of conscious thinking could override his activated stress switch in the moment. So, don't feel bad when you get worked up over something scary or have a hard time controlling your fear—even Darwin couldn't do it![34]

No one is immune to his or her stress switch, although some people are better than others at controlling it. The trick is to become aware that you're activated and turn the stress switch back off as quickly as possible, and before you do any irreparable damage, whether it be to your reputation, career, or relationships.

Prevention Strategies

Over time, you can train your stress switch to turn on less often and at lower and lower settings, and when you occasionally slide into it in worst-case scenarios, it will be for shorter amounts of time. For example, in a fight with your partner where you find you're starting to raise your voice, you will be able to recognize the signs of a stress switch flipping on, step away, and go calm yourself down. Better yet, by using that awareness alongside calming techniques such as breathing, meditation, and TouchPoints, you will learn to spot and avoid the daily landmines in your life that you know will trigger you.

I know that when I do certain things in my life, my stress switch is going to turn on. So when I have to give a forensic expert witness testimony in a capital murder trial, for example, I do things I know will calm my nervous system in advance to preempt the switch and lessen the stress effect. Being prepared ahead of time helps me keep my cortisol levels lower, which allows me to perform better and prevents the afterburn of emotional fatigue that occurs after a prolonged period of heightened stress. Afterwards, I feel better and can go about my evening as planned, rather than going home and crashing out on the couch from the prolonged stress. Ever hear the phrase, "emotionally exhausted?" That's code for the physical after-effects of excess stress.

In addition to mitigating your existing stress before going into known stressful situations, you can also use your natural avoidance patterns to help you identify situations that are likely to activate you, and then steer clear of them on purpose.

I know, for example, that cable news programs where people are fighting about politics activate my stress switch, so I don't watch them. I have no control over the things they are fighting about, so it's not worth wrecking my nervous system over it. I also refuse to feel ignorant if I don't watch people fighting for an hour about their opinions. For me, watching people who feel entitled because they are public figures to throw daggers and fight amongst themselves does not qualify as the news.

Just as we saw earlier in the social media discussion, there is always access to a rabbit hole that you can fall down, whether by watching the news, reading it, or arguing about it with strangers online. Psychologically, all these apps and news feeds and notifications are designed not to inform us of information but to keep us hooked in and watching longer.

As a parent, it's even more important to have dagger-throwing prevention strategies in place. For instance, if you allow yourself to punish your children in the moment you're upset with them, you might end up going to extremes. Before you exclaim, "That's it, you're grounded for a MONTH," remember, you're not acting smart. You already know that when you're stressed, you're going to act dumb. Your smart brain is nowhere to be found. This is an example of a dagger you throw in the heat of the moment that is so ludicrous that, once you're calm, you're going to end up regretting it and most likely reversing it. Because any right-thinking parent knows that grounding your child for a month is punishment for *you*, and if they're involved in any sports or other team activities, it's also punishment for their teammates, coaches, and more. This is why it's important to have your rules set in advance, so you're not allowing your lizard brain to cause all these problems in the moment when you're activated.

Stress Tracker

Overall, the more time you can spend in a calm state, and the less time your stress switch is on, the healthier you'll be, the better your relationships will be, and the better your life will be. So pay attention. Pay attention to when you are stressed and perpetuating stress, and use every tool you have to shift out of that whenever possible. If you are venting and this serves to fuel your anger and get someone else upset, ask yourself if it's really necessary. If you're obsessing about something that happened and you're taking it personally, ask yourself if you really want to be dealing with the situation in moments when it isn't actually happening. When you can give someone the benefit of the doubt, do it—you'll be less stressed. When your mind is making up upsetting stories about what you think someone was doing or thinking, to the extent that you are aware of what's happening, just stop it, silly, it's simply not worth it!

And if, like most people, you find that even once you've mastered noticing your stress switch, it's still an uphill battle to consciously change your responses, don't get discouraged. Seek the tools I have discussed already that work on your autonomic nervous system— EMDR, neurofeedback, TouchPoints—to reset your stress switch. Remember that conscious control is very weak when it comes to trying to control a stress switch on high. It's not that it can't work over time, which is why I'm giving you some mindful strategies. But realize using mental control tactics as the cornerstone of your stress less strategy is likely going to fall short.

Stop the Contagion

Reducing the amount of time you spend with you stress switch on subsequently reduces your chronic—and contagious—stress symptoms, and that equals lots of people being better to other people. Then, fewer daggers are likely to fly and hurt others.

In the movie *Contagion*, doctors and government officials try desperately to stop the rapid spread of a serious virus that is wreaking havoc on social order, leading to riots, looting, and other examples of the very worst of human behavior. The virus is on the verge of ruining the entire world when finally, the scientists are able to get to the bottom of things and find a cure.

We already have a contagion that's ruining the entire world, and it is stress. But since it's a far less glamorous subject, one which doesn't require ominous bright yellow outbreak suits, face shields, quarantines, and the National Guard, I doubt anyone wants to see a movie about how stress is killing us. Unfortunately, just like in the movie, disaster is playing out for millions of people every day.

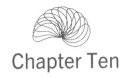

Chapter Ten

YOU'RE SO VAIN

Survival is selfish. So when you're stressed and your brain is in survival mode—you're going to act selfishly.

Lila and Caryn

Imagine this scenario: Lila and Caryn are college freshmen sharing a dorm room together. Up until now they've gotten along pretty well with no major conflicts. But there's been a storm brewing beneath the surface for Lila, who has been quietly getting more and more steamed at Caryn's general messiness. When she decided to live in a dorm with a roommate, she wasn't expecting to get paired with Oscar from *The Odd Couple*!

One day, Caryn is lying on her bunk trying to unwind after bombing a really stressful exam. The facts that she'd overslept, rushed to get ready, and arrived ten minutes late had made the event even more stressful. She can still feel her heart pounding and her thoughts are still racing.

Just as Caryn takes a few deep breaths, trying to calm herself, Lila enters the dorm room, heads to the bathroom and sees the aftermath of Caryn's chaotic morning. Beauty products and used tissues are scattered all over the counter, wet towels are on the floor, and a pile of dirty clothes sits in the corner. Unable to let the situation go on for a moment longer, Lila takes a deep breath and comes out of the bathroom to confront her sloppy roommate.

"Caryn, we need to talk, about, uh, your cleaning habits," Lila says, trying to sound diplomatic.

It's as if someone poked a hornet's nest with a stick. Caryn explodes at Lila.

"Are you KIDDING me right now? What's the MATTER with you? Can't you see I'm resting? WHY are you being so petty?"

And so on.

If Caryn's stress switch had not been activated before Lila even arrived, this conversation could be going in a whole different direction right now. The two roommates might be able stay calm, and have a rational, productive conversation about cleaning habits, maybe even setting up a cleaning schedule. But with one roommate already in a state of fight-or-flight, that is not going to happen. Although Lila started out diplomatically, Caryn has perceived the comments through a distorted lens and feels accused and attacked. With her stress switch already on, and therefore not thinking clearly, Caryn's immediate response to Lila was defensiveness.

Although it's not typically recognized as this, defensiveness is probably the most common kind of selfishness. As we saw in the example above, when someone's stress switch is on, they are more apt to respond defensively, whether they are actually being attacked or not. Defending oneself is by definition a selfish act, because the defensive person's only priority is to be right or change the other's behavior. Caryn's response, "Can't you see I'm resting?" ignores Lila's needs. Lila's reason for the initiating the conversation is not part of Caryn's equation. In stress mode we are shut down and unable to hear the other person's point of view.

Survival is an inherently selfish thing, but this is not meant to imply that selfishness is a bad thing. We need some level of selfishness in order to survive. We need to ensure that we have food, water, shelter, and clothing; and sometimes that means prioritizing our needs above other people's needs, especially if those basic needs are under threat. That's when we will lose empathy and behave selfishly.

Embedded in our moral code is an understanding that, along with the high stakes of with survival, certain otherwise selfish behaviors just come naturally. We biologically move towards protection and selfishness. For instance, we hoard resources when we feel threatened. It's been shown that adopted children tend to stockpile food in their beds. Time after time, I explain the basic survival mechanism underlying this behavior to adoptive parents in my office. A social psychology study has shown that people think it's morally okay to steal food if they or someone they love might go hungry. There's a popular ethics class parable that tells of a man who steals a loaf of bread from the store to feed his starving family. Students are asked, in light of his altruistic motive, is the stealing wrong? Might they do the same thing in his situation? The ethics discussion that ensues can go on for a while, my point is that when we are trying to survive, we will become selfish. We will defend ourselves. We will steal. We will cheat. We will ignore the needs of others. We will do these things out of necessity, and many would hesitate to label these actions selfish in such circumstances.

However, when stress puts us in a state of fight-or-flight outside of a life-or-death situation, our survival fear kicks in just the same, and our nervous system tricks us into thinking things are a matter of life-or-death. There, selfishness is created. Therefore, even when you're arguing about something relatively minor, your body might interpret it as a battle to the death. In such a state of mind, a small issue might seem to you like it will determine your identity, your ego, your place in the world around you, or your ability to control your own circumstances. All these higher-order concepts get locked together by your lizard brain in one concept: survival. The net result? You become selfish.

Getting someone whose stress switch is on to *not* be selfish is like trying to get a three-year-old to share. I laugh when we tell three-year-olds, "sharing is caring." Three-year-olds, by nature of their level of brain development, are *wired* to be selfish! Empathy does not develop until much later, so sharing is quite literally not in their neurological vocabulary.

As adults, even with well-developed empathy, it all goes out the window when our stress switch is on. Trying to bargain with someone who is activated from stress is like trying to reason with a three-year-old. They become extremely disagreeable at best, and no matter what it is you're asking, they do the equivalent of sticking out their lower lip into a pout, digging their heels into the ground, and saying, "You can't make me!" You'll be left scratching your head, wondering how it is that the grown man you married is suddenly mimicking your child, all because you asked him to take out the garbage after work (where he clearly had a bad day!).

The connection between the stress switch, empathy, and selfishness clearly translates to how people respond to requests from others, whether it's asking someone to clean up a mess at home, making the sale in business, or asking someone to donate their time or money to a non-profit organization. If the person on the receiving end of the request is in a stressful situation—for example, you catch them at the end of the day when they're trying to get out of the office and go home—they will more than likely say no. In that moment, rather than thinking about whether what you're trying to sell them could actually improve their life, or whether they could help a child in a third-world country, their stress switch is making them preoccupied with survival.

When you have tunnel vision, it's nearly impossible to be calm, empathic, giving and unselfish. Because truthfully, in that moment you are entirely self-focused, and your own internal anxiety is your priority.

Obsessive-compulsive disorder can be seen as an extreme case of the stress switch causing selfishness. Their mind is literally telling them, "If I don't ask you the same thing ten times, I'm not going to be able to continue with my day. I'm going to stay stressed. I have to deal with this first and foremost, and block everything else out, or something terrible is going to happen."

Meanwhile, as the recipient of the same question ten times, focusing on the storm outside rather than the one raging inside the person, you're thinking, "Why does this person have to keep asking this same question and bothering me? Don't they know how selfish it is to bother me like this?"

When Lila calmly asked her totally stressed out roommate for a conversation about cleaning, Caryn was stuck in tunnel vision about her test worries. Her mind was telling her, "I can't possibly talk about cleaning habits right now or give you any attention at all. If I failed that test I might not survive. My anxiety is my priority right now, and nothing else matters."

Meanwhile, as the recipient of Caryn's irrational defensiveness, and looking at a real external mess, Lila might have thought, "Why can't she open her eyes and see how selfish it is to lay around while her mess is bothering me? She is such a rude person!"

This is what's called a fundamental attribution error, meaning that when we observe other people's behaviors we more likely to assume that they are exhibiting fixed traits rather than temporary states. But when we think of ourselves and our own behavior, it is the exact opposite. We are more likely to give ourselves some slack, and believe that how we're behaving is a direct result of the temporary state we're in. Yet when we observe someone else in a stress-triggered state respond poorly, we assume it's "who they are" and become frustrated with them.

The stressed out person can't help it, though. Their stress switch is triggered, and fight-or-flight makes them very focused on protecting themselves. Outside of psychopaths or sociopaths, nobody is inherently selfish. In fact, most people are dealing with an over-reactive stress switch, and they don't know how to manage their internal anxiety any other way than to "give in" to it, and do whatever their stressed out brain demands to relieve their anxiety.

Ultimately, when dealing with someone who is in a chronic stressed out state, it's hopeless to "should" them with how *you* think they should be behaving. What is up to you is whether you're going to let their behavior activate you or not. The Serenity Prayer is a beautiful reminder of this: "God, grant me the serenity to accept the things I cannot change, the courage to change the things I can, and the wisdom to know the difference." One thing that you absolutely cannot change is how other people's nervous systems respond to stress. Your own stress response and the resulting behaviors, however, are a different story....

Venting

In one episode of the television show, *Sex and the City*, the main character Carrie goes through a painful split with her boyfriend, "Mr. Big," and ends up carrying around break-up baggage as a result of the emotional messiness. Unfortunately for her friends, Carrie dumps her mess on them in the form of talking to them about Mr. Big—incessantly. Finally, when they aren't able to take it anymore, her friends come together in an intervention of sorts and refer her to a therapist, telling her, "We need you to see a doctor because we just can't do this anymore. We love you as our friend, but we cannot be your therapists."

It's a funny episode, but with a good point: When you are venting about something stressful in your life excessively, and not within the normal short-term boundaries of, "Ugh! I had a crummy day today," what you are really doing is bringing that stress into the relationship with your friends.

There's a common misbelief that excessive venting is somehow cathartic, even healthy. People encourage it: "If you're angry, beat up on a pillow and you'll feel better," or, "If your partner cheats on you, go take it out on a punching bag."

This doesn't work. Neither does any kind of violence when you're upset work. Venting or swinging violently at an innocent object actually has the opposite effect, strengthening the neural connections around the sympathetic activation from your stress. In other words, it causes you to dig your heels in deeper, cement your upset, and lock in your selfish, stressed out, upset perspective about it.

For instance, the more Carrie vented to her friends about how *wrong* Mr. Big was in the breakup, the more her brain was memorizing, "I'm right, he's wrong, and I'm entitled to be upset about it." In turn, her body was cementing neural networks to create a memory based on that perspective, perpetuating a continual stress response around it, to the point where she literally became unable to stop obsessing about it. What she thought was normal post-break up venting was in fact keeping her in a perpetual stress loop. While Carrie Bradshaw is a fictitious character, everybody knows real people, especially women, doing this to themselves, *every day*. They are addicted to their perpetual stress loops. They just can't wait to talk to people about all the things that they're upset about—and they may not be able to think about anything else.

We've all been there. I admit that I've been guilty of this behavior in the past too, so I see both sides of the story. When it's you doing the venting, it feels like you *must* relieve this burden from your mind. You're obsessively going over what has happened, whether to make sense of it or make peace with it. You're hurting, you're upset, you're betrayed, you're angry, and you want emotional relief! You seek people to empathize with what you're going through. You want them to validate and collude with you, "taking your side" so you don't have to fight this imagined battle for survival alone. But here's the problem: as long as your stress switch is cranked up high like that, your lizard brain is running the show, and all venting does is ensure that you'll stay in this state for even longer and re-experience it more times than necessary.

When your stress switch is on in a state like this, the irony is that your health and survival may not depend on you finding yet another sympathetic ear, but rather on you finding a hack to break the loop that has you seeking the ear in the first place.

Changing Your Responses

Are you surprised at how many of the behaviors revealed in this part of the book are direct results of stress? While it's true that you can't control others' stress levels *or* how they respond to triggers, hopefully this will serve to raise *your* internal level of awareness, and help you to recognize when your *own* lizard brain has taken over— especially when you find yourself exhibiting selfish, disagreeable, almost childish behavior that can poison the pond for everyone.

When you understand that cognitive distortions, performance issues, stress-daggers, selfishness, and venting are signs of stress, you'll become more and more adept at catching yourself. And now that you know, you can practice: immediately stop what you're doing, take note, and ask yourself, "Has my stress switch turned on without my knowledge?" if you're not too deep into fight-or-flight, you will be able to dial it down, and start the process of turning your stress switch off.

The next time you realize your stress switch is on, tell yourself: "This isn't worth the damage to my nervous system," and think an alternative thought. Each time you recognize that your stress switch is on, force yourself to stop, tell yourself it's not worth it, and change your thought, you are training yourself to stop stress in its tracks. If you have TouchPoints, keep them handy so you can use them the moment you notice a trigger. Their calming effect can be more effective than trying hopelessly to consciously control your stress. And don't forget therapy, neurofeedback, and other methods like regular meditation can likely turn it around in the long run!

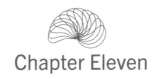

Chapter Eleven

KNEE JERKS

When you feel pressured to do something, you are more likely to make a bad decision. Stress disguises itself as a 'fear of missing out,' shuts off your thinking brain, and causes you to do things impulsively that you normally wouldn't.

When our stress switch is on and therefore our thinking brain is off, we are extremely vulnerable to impulsive behaviors, including making emotional, knee-jerk decisions. Don't think for a minute that anyone working in sales isn't completely aware of this nervous system mechanism, even if they don't know the exact mechanics. Many salespeople have specific techniques for inducing a state of stress in their client prospects, such as manufacturing a state of urgency, in order to ultimately get the person to buy their product or service. One of the best examples of this is the typical timeshare presentation.

Salespeople who give these presentations typically use time pressure as a tool to press your stress switch in the hopes that you will make an impulsive buying decision. It sounds like this: "I can't promise this price/package/location will be available tomorrow because they are in high demand," or "I'm only authorized to offer this special deal to buyers who sign up during this presentation." Because they know that if they let you go home and deliberate, first of all, you'll have time to do your research and most likely be able to deconstruct any holes in their sales pitch. Second of all, once you're removed from the excitement and anxiety of the sales situation, you'll no longer be susceptible to the impulsive behaviors that result from your stress switch being on. In other words, no sale.

When you are in the midst of situations like this it's hard for your brain to accurately distinguish the signals of excitement from anxiety. That's why the salespeople will mix together the excitement of all the great vacations you're going to have, the heartwarming, bonding family experiences, the Instagram photos that will make your friends jealous, and all the money you'll be "saving," with the anxiety of the time pressure to make a decision. You are likely to interpret the anxiety as excitement because your brain can't easily distinguish the difference between the two.

But the anxiety/excitement confusion will also contribute additional stress, possibly turning your stress switch up more. Once that salesperson gets your stress switch into the on position, you could be nearly incapable of making a clear, conscious, thinking brain decision. You'll become reactive instead of proactive and thoughtful. Your brain won't care about anything else except removing the threat and turning your stress switch off. If that means buying an overpriced, inconveniently located timeshare condo in Fiji, then so be it—it's not like your brain is going to get the bill!

That's why, when you are in a state like this, you are more likely to make an impulsive decision and exclaim with a big excited smile, "Yes, I absolutely want to do this! Sign me up!" You'll write your check and head home with visions of lounging on the beach with your family in Fiji. Then, the happy visions of sunbathing in Fiji will begin to fade when it's time to book your first vacation, and you're hit with change fees, travel fees, rental cars, getting time off from work, and other logistics, and you realize what a cumbersome operation it really is.

Adding insult to injury, once your brain is firing on all cylinders again, you might do your homework and see that you could have bought the same timeshare on the aftermarket and spent half as much. Now, you will really be regretting your impulsive decision.

Stress's impact on the brain does not bode well for decision-making, whether it's a fancy new car that's outside your budget, a risky investment choice, or a decision to leave your partner. The consequences of acting impulsively range from minor to life changing to outright life-threatening—and stress makes it worse. In an extreme case, you might be driving while incredibly stressed out and hit the gas instead of the brake. When we are in reactive stress, without access to executive brain functions, we cannot think through consequences logically and are more likely to make decisions that are not in our best interests.

Along with increased overall impulsivity, our brains crave regulation of that stress. It will signal us to engage in any behavior that brings relief, especially if the behavior has brought us relief in the past. For instance, let's say that you go shopping when you are in a state of stress and it makes you feel good temporarily. Your brain will lock in the memory that shopping relieved your stress as a positive thing. The next time you are stressed out, in order to feel a little better, your brain might unconsciously signal you to go shopping again.

This is how behavioral addictions develop—eating doughnuts, overspending, gambling, compulsively checking an app, a website, or social media, smoking, inappropriate sex, drinking too much, or doing drugs. The brain is hard-wired to memorize patterns that start when you're in a state of stress. Chronically stressed out people are more likely to give in to cravings, and their cravings are more likely to progress to addictive behaviors, all because of this impulse mechanism in the brain.

Tunnel Vision

In the timeshare example earlier, the salesperson intentionally used time pressure to manufacture an emergency situation so that he could raise anxiety and activate the stress switch, which triggered impulsive decision-making, and thus made the unsuspecting buyer (who thought they just came for a free TV) say yes to the sales pitch. The false urgency to buy became so big that the buyer lost the ability to look at the other question—did he even *want* the timeshare at all? This typifies the tunnel vision that stress causes, blocking out the full peripheral perspective of what's happening. It's easier to misgauge the actual urgency of a situation. This happened to me recently when I was getting ready to go on vacation.

Suitcases sprawled open on my bed, I darted back and forth between my bedroom and bathroom, packing for an early departure the next morning. Suddenly, there in the middle of my pre-trip chaos, a colleague texted "911," insisting that I complete some legal documents related to our business before I left. I really wanted my lawyer to have a look at the documents, but because she was insistent, my tunnel vision locked onto getting that document done. I stopped packing and, in the middle of the mess of clothes and toiletries on my bed, sat down to read.

Now under time pressure, I misread the intent of one of the clauses right off the bat. I had already been stressed out about getting everything done for my vacation, and now I was also upset about the content and implications of the paperwork I was supposed to be signing. I was unable to think clearly.

Here's where my story is different than Caryn the college freshman's story, or Carrie stuck-in-the-breakup-loop Bradshaw's story, or the poor Fijian timeshare buyer's story. First, I recognized that in my agitated state it would be really easy to make a mistake I'd regret—like throwing daggers at my colleague who was making me review a legal document instead of making sure I had my sunblock! At that moment, my efforts to practice tuning into my stress switch paid off by giving me a chance to choose something different. I could choose to take some deep breaths and try to turn my stress switch off.

Second, before my stress switch climbed from agitated all the way up to full-on fight-or-flight, I immediately put my TouchPoints on, and used the incredible tool of bilateral stimulation to shut down my tunnel vision and get back to rational thought.

As my stress levels came down, in addition to getting my peripheral vision back about the situation, I also regained the ability to think flexibly about it. I thought, "Even though I'm leaving for vacation tomorrow, it wouldn't be the worst thing if I just print out the documents, and then read them carefully and sign them on vacation. Just because someone else has unrealistic time expectations, doesn't mean it will be the end of the world if I don't adhere to them."

By recognizing that I was activated, taking measures to calm down, and then reassessing the situation outside the tunnel vision of stress, I was able to avoid a heated, potentially nasty phone call with my colleague, not to mention any binding legal consequences that would have come had I impulsively signed the documents without fully reading and understanding them.

You don't need to internalize other people's emergencies. While there are many legitimate reasons for time pressure, this is not true in all situations, and most of the time, you can choose not to buy into the urgency. As you become more and more in control of your stress levels, you'll be able to tell the difference. You'll be able to spot the impulse play, for instance, in the marketing messages on travel booking sites like, "52 people are looking at this hotel right now! Only 3 rooms left!" You'll see the artificially created time pressure, gauge where you are on the stress switch, and control your behaviors accordingly.

If you're making a decision in a state of stress, you could very well be making somebody else's decision, not your own. Whenever your stress switch is on due to any kind of pressure, time or otherwise, zooming out and taking a step back can make all the difference in the long-term outcome.

What You Can Do

What can you do if you find yourself in these pressure situations? Well first, learn to recognize what it feels like when your stress switch is on, and practice determining how high the switch has gone up. You can break this down in the following key steps.

Step One: How upset am I? The key here is to recognize your warning signs so you can identify whether your stress switch has been fully turned on. If you're not in full fight-or-flight yet, then you'll still have the conscious brainpower to act intentionally, and you can follow these steps to regain your peripheral vision in a pressure situation and make better decisions.

Step Two: Is it really urgent? If you've determined that you're not fully in fight-or-flight, take a few deep breaths and ask yourself, "Do I need to be feeling this right now? Is this really an emergency?" I'll give you a hint—if nobody's bleeding or needing to be in the hospital, it's not really an emergency. Signing that document that night was not really an emergency. If it didn't happen until the next day, no one was going to die. Take a step back from the feeling that things are your emergency when they're really a non-emergency—or someone else's emergency. Your nervous system will thank you for being able to tell the difference and not keeping it overactive unnecessarily. Your body does not want you to be stressed!

Step Three: Am I seeing everything? Next, determine if you're thinking rigidly about the situation, as in the cognitive distortion of all-or-none thinking we talked about. If you are, ask yourself how you can think and act more flexibly and create more breathing room around the situation. How can you create space between what you feel has to be done now, and seeing all your actual options?

Step Four: Pause before you decide. No matter what, try to create a pause between the thinking and the doing, so you're not making an impulsive decision in a triggered, emotional, tunnel-vision state. That is the most dangerous state from which to act.

Here's where I get to share my excitement: **if you have access to TouchPoints in the moment you realize you are stressed, there's only one step.** Turn them on and strap them on your wrists, or hide them in your pockets, socks, or tank top straps. As the bilateral stimulation calms your switch back down, you will be able to think rationally about your situation.

Anger is an especially impulsive emotion that dramatically shrinks the gap between thinking and doing. But anger can also be controlled. The common perception is that it's beyond our control, as in, "Well, I was angry. I couldn't help it. It's not my fault." But unless you are fully in fight-or-flight, you do have the capacity to create space between emotion and action. We use CBT at my clinics to teach that there is a gap between feeling anger and lashing out. If you can stay with your anger, and follow the steps above, you can create that pause and avoid consequences like broken relationships, lost jobs, injuries to yourself or others, and other often serious repercussions from acting impulsively. Creating that pause between emotion and action can be your first line of defense.

The key overall is to recognize that your stress switch is on and it's gaining momentum, catch it in the act, breathe, infuse flexible thinking, and pause before you act. Step away before hitting send on the angry email. Leave the room rather than attempting to win the argument with your partner. go home to research your buying decision rather than feeling pressured to "buy now" at the car dealership. Take a moment to calm yourself before getting behind the wheel and barreling into traffic alongside a whole bunch of other potentially stressed out drivers. Sleep on that big business decision instead of feeling obligated to make it on the spot.

In our culture we're all about actions—doing, doing, doing. We discourage pulling back from action, but when your stress switch is on, pulling back from action is oftentimes the best thing you can do. But first you need to recognize what's happening inside of you, not do something impulsive, and create the space to be able to pause. Unlike Nike, make your motto in these situations, "Just *don't* do it!"

Change of Habit

I have a friend who is a day trader who also happens to have a mother who triggers him. They have a difficult relationship and for whatever reason, he'd talk to her on Monday mornings and then, after their conversation, he'd begin day trading. With his stress switch turned on by the call (sometimes a lot!), he would be so upset that he'd make bad day trading decisions that would have a negative effect on him financially.

I suggested that a simple schedule change could help break this pattern of bad decision-making that happened whenever his stress switch was on. Knowing that he did yoga anyway on Wednesdays, I suggested that instead of doing his trading on Mondays after he talked to his mom, he might do it on Wednesdays after he did yoga. This one small change absolutely made a difference for my friend. Following his yoga practice, he was calm instead of agitated, and his stress switch was completely off. Therefore, not surprisingly, he made better day trading decisions. You can plan your life in a way that avoids pairing known stressful activities with important decision making.

There's a concept called keystone habits that says changing just one habit can create a cascade of ideally better, more positive habits. If you know you have a hectic commute to work, rather than arriving at the office and jumping right into high-pressure situations and making important decisions, you can plan to take a few minutes first to step away and decompress. Create space and in doing that, break your pattern.

Your results will be so much better if you make an effort to be calm when you face high-stakes conversations. If you are stuck in traffic that has you frustrated and activated, then picking up the phone while you drive to have a chat with your partner about a touchy topic is not a good decision. I guarantee that in a triggered state, you will *not* resolve the touchy topic, and if the conversation doesn't go well, you've now increased the chances that if someone cuts you off in traffic, you'll go into road rage. The individual decisions and choices you make, especially in situations where you *know* you're likely to be activated, have the power to better or worsen the kinds of life situations that many people believe are out of their control. It's up to you to take responsibility for seeing the pattern and then rework it as needed.

If you have a row of dominoes set up a certain way, pushing down the first one inevitably pushes down the others in the same pattern every single time. If you know that ahead of time, and you don't want that last domino to fall where it does, you'll rearrange the line in a different way to avoid that outcome. If you know that a certain trigger stresses you, and when you're stressed you're prone to bad decision-making, then rearrange your pattern to create a space between stress and big decisions. Be smart about the things that you *do* know and modify your habits based on that knowledge! With awareness, there are many more things in life within your control than you might believe.

The bottom line about habits and stress is that when you're stressed is *not* the time to be making important decisions if you can avoid it. Be aware of the signs that someone is trying to set off your emergency stress switch when there's really no emergency. Create any pauses you can between your anger and impulsive outward expressions of it. When in doubt, sit on it. You want to draft a scathing email when you're mad? Go ahead—but put yourself on the address line so you can't impulsively send it to anyone else. And for the past moments when you didn't do these things, forgive yourself, because you didn't know any better. Resolve to do better next time. Beating yourself up certainly will not move your stress switch in the right direction. So be calm and carry on....

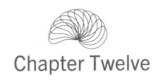

Chapter Twelve

NEGATIVE PREDICTIONS

It is important to distinguish between stress itself and the events that can cause stress. Stress is an internal state. Stressors are the triggers that happen to us which cause the various levels of stress that we've all experienced in our lives.

My boyfriend was going through a rough patch. At work, he'd lost a big account. At home, he'd overheard me arranging a work dinner with somebody I used to date. His stressors bred stressors of my own when his stress switch ratcheted up high enough to set off some childish exchanges, and one thing led to another. One night, I asked him to wake me the next morning—and he did not. I was jarred awake by the doorbell: one notch up on my own switch. Clock said I was late: notch number two. I tracked him down in the house and confronted him, impulsively. He said he forgot. Already activated, I concluded my boyfriend was lying to me: notch number three.

"Why didn't you wake me?" I snapped at him, throwing daggers.

"It's not my job to wake you up. I'm not your employee!" He got defensive. Bad news.

"But you *said* you were going to wake me up!" Defensive *and* accusatory.

It only escalated from there, as you might imagine, the stress sucking completely unrelated trigger points from our relationship into our conversation. Have you ever been there?

I later called that our "TouchPoints moment" of the month. If either or both of us had been wearing our TouchPoints that morning, the whole ugly scene might never have happened. But in the moment, fight-or-flight was in full effect on both sides, and it did not go well.

Once the argument was over and we'd retired to our separate corners, my stress-addled lizard brain spun off a whole barrage of questions like, "Oh my gosh, are we compatible? Do I break up with him? Is this what he's really like? Can I deal with this for the long-term?" My irrational brain (from my stress switch being on) had managed to turn a harmless argument about oversleeping into a paranoid frenzy about potentially breaking up with my boyfriend whom I love very much! This special kind of harmful thought is also a side effect of an unchecked stress switch: they are called negative predictions.

The future looked dire because I was lost in a mercury-filled pond of cognitive distortions with no filter to differentiate reality from fantasy. My stressors had me spinning in circles.

Negative Predictions

You have an inner fortune-teller, and let me tell you, she is a fickle character, completely inconsistent. When your stress switch is off, your fortune-teller is a unequivocally positive, optimistic best friend—the one that tells you everything you want to hear and wants you to live your best life. She whispers in your ear about all the wonderful things that are going to happen to you. On top of that, even when the not-as-wonderful things come along, she tells you that everything will be alright. You've got this. You can handle anything that comes your way. Life is good, and you are sittin' pretty!

When your stress switch is on, however, your fortune-teller takes on a whole new personality—the hag! Now she's whispering all the bad things that can potentially happen. She's also telling you that *when* (not if) those bad things do come along, you won't have what it takes to handle them. You will crumble under the pressure. That mean old hag, brought to life by your stressors, feeds on all things horrible and is powered by catastrophic thinking.

This hag, of course, is nothing more than a collection of stories inside your head. Whether the stories you're telling yourself are positive or negative depends on where your nervous system is aligned. When you're calm, your nervous system tells your brain to believe the positive stories. When you're stressed, your brain believes the negative ones—and uses them to support negative predictions about your future. When you believe these negative predictions as reality, you are likely to act out of fear and reap the consequences of what is nothing more than a nervous system hallucination.

Remove the stress, and your executive brain recalibrates your mental filter. The happy, positive fortune teller returns, gently wipes away the cognitive distortions that the hag used to muddy your thinking, and reminds you, "You know what? You don't really know what the future holds!"

Pessimism vs. Negative Predictions

Negative predictions and pessimism are not the same thing. Pessimism afflicts the person who chooses to chronically listen to their inner hag. They accept her lies of, "This will never work... this bad thing will surely happen... and what if this other bad thing happens next?" as gospel, and live their life accordingly. Pessimists smother themselves in excessive "what ifs," predict that all things won't go well, and are preparing for the worst at all times. While pessimism is an overall negative attitude—one that can be shifted, by the way—negative predictions are connected directly to the state of your nervous system, and fluctuate based on where you are on the stress switch.

Thinking positively instead doesn't mean that everything will always turn out well for you, but what it does do is free up the time leading up to potentially negative events. Rather than fueling a chronically triggered state with negative predictions, being optimistic allows you to enjoy the time before the event thinking and feeling positively, while a pessimist might have wasted it in a state of stressed out dread. You can even prepare for the very worst without being in a stressed out state too. There are ways to prepare for the unexpected, without staying in a constant negative state. This is why we have insurance, contracts, and lawyers! If you are thinking positively and something doesn't turn out well, you handle it and move on.

As I'm writing this, my house is under contract to sell. I think the inspection will come back okay, the buyers will not back out of the deal, and the sale will go well. And if that doesn't happen, there is a clause in the contract that says that the buyers will owe me money— so I'm covered either way. That's a way to prepare for the worst without being stressed. I refuse to let the hag take over and needlessly flip my stress switch on for the whole time leading up to closing. It's just not worth it.

Negative appraisals of life, especially chronic ones, impact more than peace of mind. Contributors to chronic stress, they also can threaten your job, hurt your family dynamics, and ruin entire relationships.

In a way that is similar to our stress switches, we all have a pessimism-optimism scale, and a baseline along that scale that we tend towards when we're calm. We shift away from our baseline based on our overall stress level, and in response to any kind of mental or physical stressor. I certainly have more negative predictions when I have PMS than I do when not. I'm fully aware that a situation that's stressing me out while I have PMS would produce far fewer negative predictions a week later. But in those hormonally charged, stressed out moments, it's hard for me to see outside of my stress snow globe. I know that I have to take extra steps to stay calm and be positive during those times of the month because my neural chemistry is working against me.

The amount of stress you're carrying around at any given time helps determine whether your inner fortune-teller is optimistic about what life has in store for you, or if she's convinced that your life sucks and you're going to die. The great news is that *you* are responsible for your stress level and for recognizing the cognitive distortions high stress causes, including negative predictions.

Stressor Rankings

Not all stress is created equal. A major reason that real estate transactions are incredibly stressful for most people is that shelter is a core, primal human need. When you move, you're uprooting your shelter, your possessions, and your basic sense of security.

The Holmes and Rahe stress scale is a list of the top psychological stressors people can experience in life, and a change in living conditions ranks high in the top forty. At the top of the list are death of a partner, divorce, marital separation, imprisonment, death of a close family member, personal injury or illness, marriage, dismissal from work, marital reconciliation, retirement, change in health of a family member, pregnancy, sex difficulties, gaining a new family member, business readjustment, and a change in financial state. Every individual will process these external stressors differently depending on their stress switch baseline. Each of these storms within will have its own shape and weight based on the person's ACEs, stress coping mechanisms, and other individual factors; and the Holmes and Rahe model predicts that someone experiencing just two or three of these events in a 12-month period may have a 50 percent chance of a health breakdown in the following two years.[35] But across the board, any major life change can bring out the hag and her dark cloud of negative predictions. The more external life stressors you're dealing with, the more negative predictions your brain will make. It is important to be aware of this connection so you can prepare in advance and hopefully even catch that nasty hag in the act of cranking your stress switch even higher.

When my children visit their father overseas, not only do I expect to be stressed about my children being out of the country, but I also know my hag will come out and try to make negative appraisals about my business, my body image, my relationship, and all the other areas of my life. When that stress switch is turned on, she can be ruthless!

How we think about our lives, our relationships, and ourselves fluctuates from moment to moment along with our nervous system activity. Having and acting on that knowledge is a lot better than flying blindly, shooting daggers at others, reaping the repercussions, and living at the mercy of your nervous system.

Exaggerated Predictions

We can make some predictions based on past behavior, like my friend who says that nine times out of ten, on Fridays you can find her ex drinking at a bar. Since this has been true in the past, the probability is pretty high that she's correct. But at the same time, the stress she feels while talking about it will moderate her prediction. In reality, her ex might not go to that bar *every* Friday, but her experience when they were together was that he always did, and it stressed her out. Because of that, her brain may overestimate the frequency of this event; and further, she may make distorted negative predictions that he's getting wasted, that he's getting in trouble, he's driving drunk, and is a threat to others. In reality, maybe he's going out a couple times a month after work, having a couple of beers with some friends, and going home.

Certain processes embedded in our society support our tendencies to make exaggerated predictions. A few years ago I was drafting legal documents. My lawyer managed to trigger some stress with a slew of worst-case scenarios about everything that could go wrong that I needed to consider. Based on *his* fear-based negative predictions, he created all kinds of scary possibilities for me to consider.

It's a lawyer's job to plan for every possible catastrophe, and they understand better than anyone all the ways people can be taken advantage of in legal situations. But he created a very stressful dynamic and a lot of fear inside of me. For a short period of time, I allowed my inner hag to turn my lawyer's professional efforts to protect me into negative exaggerations and worrying when, in fact, nothing bad was happening. As I became aware of my growing activation, I made myself pause to breathe, and I reminded myself that the chance of those catastrophic possibilities actually happening was slim-to-none. I lowered my stress switch.

It's inevitable, through the laws of probability, that some negative predictions will come true. But that doesn't mean it's your job to stay on high alert, living in a continual state of stress, constantly on the lookout for validation that life sucks or will certainly suck tomorrow or the next day. Don't fall victim to cognitive distortions that can wrongly validate your negative predictions. If you're seeking the hag, looking for the negative, of course it will be visible all around you, especially if you're in a stressed out state to begin with. Anxiety is not a security blanket or insurance against bad things happening to you. All it does is ensure your misery while you wait for bad things to show up, and it sows dangerous health consequences in the meantime, for you to reap later.

Thwarting Danger

At my clinics, we work with law enforcement officers who have been in critical incidents where they've been shot or their partners have been shot or killed. Many of them develop PTSD if they don't get treatment right away. And many have PTSD before they even encounter critical incidents due to the high stress of the job.

I worked with one officer who had been called to testify against the criminals who had shot him and killed his partner. Planning to go to court was incredibly stressful, because not only would my client have to testify while he was grieving, but he would have to listen to these criminals essentially tell lies for two hours.

As I was preparing him for the experience, this very honorable, kind, heroic man, who had survived an awful experience on the job, wasn't sure he'd be able to control himself in court. He confided, "Doc, I'm afraid I'm going to hurt someone. I'm really afraid I'm going to get so upset and angry that I'm going to stand up, walk across the courtroom, lose my mind, and assault somebody." Here was a good man, not a violent one, who was angry, grieving the death of his partner, and who was suffering from PTSD and terribly afraid of losing control.

No matter what perceptions and opinions you have about police officers as a whole, I will tell you that in a situation like this, there is usually no wrongdoing by law enforcement. These are good men. Every police officer has to go through psychological testing to ensure they're sane before they join an agency. But after ten or fifteen years on the job, their psychological profiles can look much different as a result of the job. Oftentimes people don't take that into consideration.

This was an honest, sane police officer who had gone through a terrible tragedy, and his negative predictions that he might attack the defendants were direct effects of his PTSD. As we talked in my office before the trial about that, I put TouchPoints on him and told him to keep thinking about those negative predictions, and how he might harm the defendants in the courtroom. After he had worn the TouchPoints for a couple of minutes, I asked him how he was feeling.

"I think I'm calmer," He said. "I feel better. I feel like if I have these, I may not get so upset, and I feel like I can control myself."

His new prediction turned out to be absolutely right. He used his TouchPoints before, during, and after his appearance on the witness stand, first holding them in his hands whenever he thought about the trial, and then, in court, tucking them into his socks. Sure, he got upset while he was in the courtroom facing the men who shot him and murdered his partner; he's a human being. But the bilateral tactile stimulation from the TouchPoints kept his stress switch down on low and kept his brain out of fight-or-flight mode, and everyone in the courtroom stayed safe.

Mental Rehearsals

Consider this: when you make negative predictions, you're mentally rehearsing something negative happening in your life, which can then carry over to your behavior and actions, and increase and the likelihood that you will make those predictions reality. Stress is like the director of a constantly running stage play in your mind, in which bad things are constantly happening to the actors!

Even an accurate prediction can be exaggerated into something more menacing and out-of-control when stress is introduced into the equation. A minor fear of public speaking can turn into full-blown fight-or-flight mode when someone's stress switch is already on.

Barry

Barry, a top executive at his company, told me the day before he was to give a big speech at work, "Every time I have a speaking engagement at work, my hands start to shake, my chest gets flushed,

I start bumbling around for what to say, and I feel like an idiot. I just know that's what's going to happen tomorrow." He blamed this usual reaction—and his lifetime of negative predictions around public speaking—on a humiliating childhood experience speaking in front of the class.

Before I could do any active treatment on him, he had to give the presentation. When he came back, he said, "Guess what happened? I gave my presentation and my hands shook, and my chest got flushed, and I bumbled around for what to say, and I felt like an idiot." Of course he did. Barry's unchecked stress levels practically guaranteed that his negative predictions would become a self-fulfilling prophecy.

Before coming to see me, Barry had tried to outsmart his anxiety; to talk himself out of automatically sliding into the panicked state whenever speaking in front of a group. The "power of positive thinking" is a popular idea right now. We want to think that it is possible to use positive thinking to counteract distorted negative predictions. But remember, you can't trick your nervous system. Your nervous system believes it understands threats far better than you do. You may be thinking, "Silly brain, calm down, I'm just trying to give a sales presentation here!" But, when the excess stress in your body has the stress switch on, your brain argues back, "Uh-uh, I have it on good authority that we are under ATTACK!!!" You can get away with some lies in life, but you cannot lie to your brain. It's like someone telling you there's no fire when the alarm in the building is blasting loud and clear.

Barry had tried positive affirmations, but his stress activation was much too high for them to be effective. But in treatment, he learned that stress and related conditions like negative predictions are not forever states. Moment-to-moment fluctuations on our stress switch dictate our body's responses and behaviors. When we change the fluctuations, we change the behaviors. Once we treated his unchecked stress levels, his fight-or-flight reaction to public speaking ceased. In Barry's case, this meant going from panicked to cool, calm, and collected while presenting. His relentless negative prediction that he would have to live with this reaction forever was also eliminated. The hag in our head does her best to convince us that stress and the hallucinations it causes are permanent. But we are not and we are helpless to change.

Negative Appraisals

Negative appraisals are a broader form of negative predictions that take the form of critical and unkind lies your brain tells you about yourself.

John

John, a seventy-year-old EMDR therapy patient, was ridiculed incessantly as a child because of a physical visual impairment. Even though the problem has been long corrected, he still feels like that little boy with low self-esteem, cowering in the face of constant teasing, and feeling very negative about himself.

John had been living in negative appraisals about himself for decades, beating himself up mentally the way the children in school used to beat him up for his physical disability. The low self-esteem from his childhood caused a pattern of unchecked chronic stress that led to negative appraisal after negative appraisal, which have impacted his self-worth, behaviors, and actions for most of his life. His inner hag makes up lies about him that he has believed without question as the truth. She's constantly telling him, "Oh, you're just a little maimed boy that isn't worth anything."

He has built a successful business and made millions of dollars selling a product that helps people, is a good husband and family man, and by external standards, an absolute success. But meanwhile, internally, John has lived a tortured life in a constant state of stress, because he can't believe any of the good things that are true about himself or his life.

During his EMDR treatment with me the fog of chronic stress slowly lifted. In one session, he suddenly had an awakening and asked, "Wait.... Why did I think for so many years that I wasn't worthy? I was the number one salesperson in my company for *years*. And then I became an entrepreneur and did all these great things..." He stumbled. "But I picked an abusive business partner..."

And then he paused as he realized, "Wait a second! That's because I actually needed capital at that point, and he came in with capital and made it sound easy. There were good reasons why I picked him."

With his stress lifted, he was finally able to see that and stop beating himself up for what he'd thought was a terrible decision. Balanced thinking only came in once his stress switch was dimmed. While he acknowledged that he would have preferred a partner with better character, he could also see the good reasons for the decision at the time.

Negative Health Predictions

The storm John had experienced was not limited to his internal mental state, either. That level of stress over such a length of time inevitably affected his physical health too.

Your beliefs are powerful. Negative thinking can cause inflammation in your body. A chemical cascade happens with negative thoughts, which doesn't occur the same way with positive thoughts. But you can't trick yourself with positive thoughts, especially positive thoughts that you don't believe in—they don't work. You need to remove the stress that is triggering those thoughts.

When John said, "I'm just worthless," and I told him, "No, you're not. You're amazing," he couldn't assimilate that; his activated stress switch wouldn't let him believe good things about himself. But once we treated the root, chronic nervous system activation triggering these false beliefs, he was finally able to see that he is a good person, he has done good things in his life that have helped many people, and that none of those old negative appraisals are true. When evidence is presented that is contrary to the negative thought, the negative appraisals begin to dissolve.

A recent study revealed that if a person combined a pre-existing medical condition with a high stress level that they perceived as unmanageable, their medical condition was more likely to get worse, as well as their mortality rate. This was in contrast to the individuals who were either able to manage their stress, or saw it as not a big issue.[36]

In another study, "Positive Emotions in Early Life and Longevity," researchers collected handwritten autobiographies from 180 Catholic nuns who were an average of twenty-two years old, scored their biographies for emotional content, and then looked at their survival rate between ages seventy-five and ninety-five. They found that the women who had exhibited more positive emotions in their writing at age twenty-two had longer lifespans than the women whose writing had reflected less positivity. Then they correlated those emotional scores with a variety of factors like gender, nutrition, social support, and medical care, and posited that while longevity is related to all those combined factors, positivity alone plays a significant role. The finding that how these nuns expressed themselves in their journals could predict their mortality rate is extremely revealing.[37]

Similar findings have been seen about which cancer patients survive and which do not. Useful predictors of cancer survival rate go far beyond the type of cancer and treatment to include a whole host of other factors, including social support, the patient's perception of their diagnosis, the positive, healthy behaviors they engage in, and other subjective influences.

Something to consider here is the way that a negative appraisal of yourself and life is likely to cause less healthy behaviors like poor nutrition, lack of exercise, alcohol consumption, and addictions, all of which cause inflammation and sympathetic activation, and thus require nervous system regulation.

We can see how this works if we examine common attitudes about success in dieting. An optimistic dieter will think, "Dieting has been hard, but if I put my mind to it, I think I can succeed. It may be slower progress than I want, but it's still worth a shot." Therefore, when faced with temptation, like a fast food drive-thru, they'll probably keep driving. This type of attitude avoids all-or-nothing thinking by acknowledging that slow progress *is* progress.

But the pessimistic dieter will think, "Well, I'm not going to lose that much weight, anyway. It's too hard, so I'm going to pig out on fast food!" Once the fast food is in hand, that person's hag will show up and announce, "Well, you just blew your diet completely. You suck at this, so you might as well just eat like crap for the rest of the day. You're never going to lose this weight now, so you might as well have fun!" The hag distorts a small setback into a complete failure, and uses it to support an irrationally negative prediction, which gives them a license to quit. That is all-or-nothing thinking in a nutshell, Now, to compound the stress, they're emotional and depressed, setting off a further negative cycle of behaviors and actions.

The key to disrupting negative cycles of behavior like this lies within your consciousness. You must raise your awareness of how much your stress switch is turned on. Learn to observe yourself: are you calm, rational, and thinking positively? Or are you stressed out, irrational, and thinking negatively, and thus engaging in behaviors that you know aren't good for you? In this way, positive thinking absent of stress-induced negative predictions leads to better overall health. When you learn to first be aware of and then regulate these fluctuations along the stress switch, you will make better and ultimately healthier decisions, physically and emotionally.

And there's more good news. How you handle stress can create spontaneous changes. Electroencephalogram data has shown that using TouchPoints changes brain wave activity associated with negative thinking—so thoughts may spontaneously become more positive while using them.

Negative Predictions on a Larger Level

When people have a polarized viewpoint, whether at the citizen-, politician-, or world leader-level, they're likely to get activated when someone introduces a conflicting viewpoint or worse, acts on it. When their stress switch gets triggered this way, negative predictions can kick in; this explains why some people react as though Armageddon is imminent when someone contradicts their point of view: "The stock market is going to crash! This is Hitler all over again! Communism is around the corner! The nuclear bombs will start falling any minute now!"

These kinds of overblown, negative predictions are rampant in the media and social media, and like other stress behaviors, when they take hold they are very contagious. In an activated state, many people absolutely believe that these negative predictions, no matter how farfetched and catastrophic, will happen.

Now imagine if, before they got wrapped up in this cycle, each individual had an awareness of their stress switch, and made the choice to consciously control it? How could that level of personal responsibility for stress and how it affects others shift our inherent make-up as a culture and a country? Would it be possible to change the behavior of a nation by changing the behavior of the individuals within it?

On an individual level, how much are you willing to let other people's negative appraisals of the world, of themselves, and of others (including you) dictate how you live your life? How much will you allow your stress switch to be turned on by others, and then live with the consequences? It's up to you.

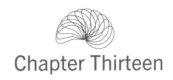

Chapter Thirteen

GOING OFFLINE

Humans now have access to an artificial world where we can connect to devices rather than people, and be in artificial light twenty-four hours per day. Our bodies simply aren't designed for this. The result is circadian rhythm disruption and sleep deprivation that threatens our performance, cognition, health, and can even be deadly.

(Spoiler alert: If you haven't already seen the movie *Fight Club* and intend to, skip this part.) In the movie, the main character's overwhelming insomnia makes him hallucinate a whole other personality (in the form of Brad Pitt) and create an entirely new storyline of his life driven by the hallucinated Pitt's erratic actions. His sleep-deprived hallucinations are a constant state of extreme fight-or-flight (mostly fight, as the movie's title reflects), and he believes it's all real. He believes this until the end of the story, when his life is in ruins and nearly ended by the actions of his alternate ego, and he realizes he has imagined the whole thing.

Fight Club is a fictitious and extreme example of the very real effects of sleep deprivation, but the moral of the movie and our own stories as human beings in the real world is the same: lack of sleep can be deadly, not only to your body, but to your relationships, all the other areas of your life, and to your potential as a human being.

Even one night of impaired sleep can significantly alter your intellectual functioning, your motor control, and sway your mood to irritable, moody, anxious, and depressed. Just one night and you're more likely to make mistakes at work, and you're more likely to get in a car accident. At the level of chronic sleep deprivation, your neurochemistry becomes dysregulated, preventing you from functioning normally—physically, emotionally, and mentally. No part of you is spared. Without enough quality sleep, you are at best an incomplete, out-of-focus version of yourself, and at worst, you're a walking-dead zombie! Regulating your sleep is a vital part of your overall strategy to stay calm, focused, productive, and healthy.

Dysregulated

Barring any severe medical conditions, some people are sleep-dysregulated by choice. The teenager that decides to be on Snapchat and play video games until 2 A.M. every night. The late-night party animal who seems to come to life only when the sun goes down, and the student who pulls all-nighters for exams are all examples of people *consciously* choosing to dysregulate their sleeping patterns. Whether they know it or not, they're choosing to not be at the top of their game by increasing the possibility of making more mistakes in their waking life. Their choice will start moving their stress switch from low to high, making it more and more difficult for them to be calm in their daily life. They'll be more easily triggered, and by things that normally would not trigger them at all. And therefore they will spend more and more time in fight-or-flight, sowing the seeds for long-term health consequences.

Sometimes the choice to wake up early or go to bed late is not simply a choice. In his bestselling book, *Why We Sleep*, Matthew Walker describes two basic sleep profiles—those who are hard-wired to wake up early in the morning, and night owls. I can see the light bulbs popping up over the heads of my fellow parents out there, who have one child who wakes up naturally at 5 A.M. every day, no matter when they go to bed, and another who has a hard time falling asleep, stays awake late, and has to be dragged out of bed at 9 A.M. According to Walker, a true night owl may not become dysregulated by late hours the way an early riser would. Their DNA may be hard-wired to go to bed later and wake up later. The key there is to also wake up later—the night owl is not more resistant to sleep *deprivation*, nor to the impairments it causes. Unfortunately, our job structures and school systems aren't exactly structured around the night owl's sleep patterns, so the end result is often chronic deficiency at one end or the other, which can create dysregulation and stress.

Through it all though, sleep is a natural thing. Your body wants to sleep; your brain needs sleep; it's a matter of survival. If it's not happening, then for whatever reason there's something off, and that's going to wreak havoc on every single system in your body over time. Sleep is the ultimate body regulator, and when it becomes dysregulated, your entire state as a human being is threatened.

Stress and Sleep

There are other, often serious, medical conditions that can cause insomnia. However, the predominant reason most people have trouble with sleep is stress. You don't need to be in a state of bliss to fall asleep, but you do need to be reasonably calm, without incessant mind chatter amping you up.

Not only can you not fall asleep when your stress switch is on, but stress also makes it unlikely you'll be able to stay asleep, because your body, in all its hyper-vigilance, will wake you back up. The two most common problems I see are difficulty falling asleep and difficulty staying asleep for the recommended seven to nine hours of sleep every night.

I treat a lot of sleep issues in high-strung people who run their brain at full speed from the moment they wake up until the moment they go to bed. The barrage of thoughts and worries that their brain processes on a daily basis would be enough to crash the world's highest bandwidth computer. They don't allow themselves any quiet moments for their brain to acknowledge and deal with their thoughts, to rest, and to shut down. Their nervous system runs amok in a constant state of activation. The stress they believe they're managing during the day turns into an outright neurological power struggle at night. And this struggle includes not only the stress they're aware of, but also any hidden issues.

Sleep can be an accurate diagnostician of life events that you think you're handling well but are really not, including past traumas you thought you'd handled already, but still need to process. Allowing stress to build up in your mind all day is like shoving a whole bunch of clothes, paperwork, knick-knacks and other things you don't want to deal with into a closet. Bag after bag, you push it all into the closet, hoping it's a magic closet, and everything will somehow vanish once it's in there. Eventually, it gets harder and harder to shut the door, but you lean into it until it closes. Finally, at the end of the day, unable to contain its contents any longer, the closet door bursts open, and all that stuff comes rushing out, making a mess of your whole house. That's what it's like when you let all your stressful thoughts build up all day, refusing to deal with them. When you finally do try to power down your brain, the door comes flying off and all those thoughts and worries flood into your consciousness.

Meanwhile, it's bedtime, so you're trying to will yourself to sleep with a few deep breaths and a command: "Okay brain—relax!" But your brain says, "Are you kidding me right now?" and you spend another sleepless night tossing and turning in bed, staring at your alarm clock as the worry reel in your brain plays a nonstop loop.

You'll always be unsuccessful at ordering your brain to relax. That's not at all how relaxation works. Relaxation requires letting go, not more control. It's not another task to delegate to your already overactive brain. Not everything requires hard work or the overly complicated processes that you've repeatedly tried to inflict on your brain. Actions, even mental ones, put your brain into motion towards a specific, intended result. Relaxation and sleep operate in the exact opposite way. They require releasing action items, rather than adding more for your mind to do. They require not trying to jam more stuff into the closet.

Your ability to relax and let go at bedtime is directly related to how you handle all those thoughts that came up during the day. Did you deal with them as they came up, or did you shove them into the closet, so that the garbage comes flooding into your brain just as you're trying to sleep? It can be completely overwhelming to be confronted by every thought, worry, and negative prediction the day produced, all at the same time, and at the worst possible time, too!

A better way is to clean up your thoughts as they happen by first becoming aware of each thought and then acknowledging that it can be changed. Also, bring awareness to how you feel physically during the thought—where does it put your stress switch on the spectrum between on and off? Does the thought make your heart race? Breathe more quickly? Give you a stomachache? A headache? By now you know what all that means; it means you're in fight-or-flight, and you'll need to handle that first. Before you have any hope of talking yourself out of a troublesome thought, you'll need to bring your stress switch back down, through breathing, meditation, TouchPoints, or whatever else you've found that works.

When your rational thinking returns, you'll be able to see that it's just a thought, you don't have to believe it, and if there's associated action to be taken, you have a choice: do it immediately or delegate it for later, rather than cramming it in the closet and wasting your time with worry in the meantime.

It will help if you can begin to build a self-management system for dealing with thoughts and worries the moment they come up, rather than continuously stuffing them away so they inevitably come flooding into your head at bedtime. Acknowledge thoughts, check your stress level, bring yourself out of fight-or-flight as needed, realize the thought itself is not a threat, take action on it or schedule it for later, and move on.

Your Stress Switch Scale

Your ability to dim your stress switch back down depends on how high it is turned up. Here is a guide you can use to self-assess your stress switch level. The guide will also make it clear why, when your switch is up in the higher numbers, it is much more difficult (or impossible) to dim it back down on your own using methods like happy thoughts, deep breathing, and yoga. The higher your switch is, the more firmly your sympathetic nervous system is in control. And remember, a nervous system problem requires a nervous system solution.

0   When your stress switch is off, you are calm and focused, have the ability to access joyful thoughts and higher-order thinking skills, gain new insights, and feel connected to things outside of yourself.

1-3   Under mild stress, you will still have the ability to notice stress-related feelings and thoughts and very likely, be able to use conscious thoughts to lower your switch. You probably won't have stress-related body sensations happening at this level.

4-6   Disturbing body sensations like chest tightness, mild muscle tension, and some increase in heart and breathing rates are a sign that your stress switch is climbing to this level. These physical symptoms alone happen at a level far below a state of full-blown fight-or-flight; you will have some ability to notice this state and attempt to use conscious thoughts or breathing techniques to bring it down.

7-8   If your stress switch has climbed to this level, you will become behaviorally unreasonable, unable to process verbal information accurately or use cognitive strategies. In other words—you won't be able to think clearly. Here, you may recognize your disordered thinking, but beware: at this level, you lose the ability to "outwit" your stress with conscious thoughts. You will need a nervous system disruptor (like TouchPoints or EMDR therapy, for instance) to bring your stress switch down for you.

9-10   Full-blown fight-or-flight mode is easily identifiable by the presence of dramatic physical effects like racing heartbeat; shallow, rapid breathing; and chest tightness (although it is possible for these symptoms to be absent, or to go unnoticed, in fight-or-flight mode). Mentally and emotionally, you will be a reactive mess.

The data I've analyzed from the TouchPoint Challenge, which we've administered on tens of thousands of people, shows that just *one stressful thought* can elevate someone's stress switch to a 7 or 8 on the scale.[38] Think about that for a moment. It doesn't take an actual life-threatening physical emergency; just one thought can take a person nearly to full-blown fight-or-flight syndrome! This means that, while conventional methods like deep breathing, yoga, and meditation can be your go-to methods for moments when your stress switch is on at level 1-6, they are simply not a complete strategy. The fact that the stress switch gets turned on so high and so quickly for many people reveals why conventional methods of stress relief have failed us so far—especially in extreme situations.

Going to Extremes

When someone has a problem with sleep on a regular basis, it manifests in a similar way to panic. One of the hallmarks of panic disorder is the fear of future panic attacks, and worse, negative predictions that the attacks may never end. When someone has a panic attack, the fear of having another panic attack prolongs it. The same happens with insomnia. After a couple of terrible nights, the stress of the sleeplessness combines with the foggy thinking caused by sleep deprivation to produce catastrophic and negative predictions like, "What if I can't fall asleep? What if I never sleep again? What if it's like this forever for me?" The stress of that thought cycle then keeps the person awake for more nights, escalating into a self-fulfilling prophecy. Now a couple of terrible night's sleep really can develop into a chronic inability to relax the brain and body into a state of sleep.

This pattern happens overall with chronic stress, too. When a person doesn't find relief from a single incident of stress, the stress of not finding relief creates more stress, and suddenly the person is left wondering if they'll ever be unstressed again. The negative hag in their head shows up and assures them they will not.

In stress and sleep cycles like this, the mind is altered and cognitive distortions can run rampant, blurring the lines of perception so that solvable problems can seem hopeless and turn an otherwise clear-headed, reasonable person into a shell of their former self.

Remedies

The most often-prescribed solution to sleep disorders is a sleeping pill. When people take sleeping pills, they will get a sufficient number of hours of sleep, but still report waking up feeling groggy, and often have negative side effects from the drug itself. The goal should be to use solutions with as few side effects or consequences as possible, but many sleep medications are at the exact opposite end of that spectrum.

In my clinic, we use medications as one mode of treatment, but pharmaceuticals are not part of our regular practice for treating people with sleep disorders. In almost all the cases we've had over the last ten years, we've been able to get people regulated and improve the quality of their sleep using methods other than sleeping pills. Here are some of those methods.

Avoiding Artificial Light at Night

When I was consulting with a group working in Africa, a group of well-meaning workers were proud to be involved in a project that would mean the local power grid would not longer turn off at eight o'clock every night. The workers were so excited to bring people 24-7 access to technology, light, and other life conveniences needing power. My reaction when they told me about this surprised them.

"Uh-oh..." I said, frowning.

"Uh-oh what?" one of the workers said, anxious about my reaction.

"Once you start adding light at night past a certain point, you're risking a whole group of new potential problems stemming from circadian rhythm dysregulation that this population is at all used to. Things like obesity, anxiety, depression, mental health disorders, and early menstruation in young girls."

The workers were surprised and I could tell a little upset to hear this. "Wait a minute, Dr. Serin!" They protested, "What you're saying doesn't sync with what we know about electricity, at all. We thought power was a GOOD thing!"

Electricity is a good thing. But exposure to artificial light past when the sun goes down is *not* good for us as organisms. As soon as the sun goes down, our body should begin neurochemically preparing for sleep. Artificial light effectively hijacks that process by suppressing the production and release of melatonin, especially when you need it most, at bedtime. Even if you're getting the recommended seven to nine hours of sleep most nights, any artificial light at all in your sleep environment can still take away from the quality of your sleep.

Let's first set the record straight on artificial light and what it is, as this appears to be a source of confusion for many people. Many believe that by having the display setting on their phone and other devices switch from "daytime" to "nighttime" they've solved the problem. Voilà. No more artificial light!

But the screen on your devices, as I pointed out to the workers in Africa, is only one source of problematic light. The "blue light" theory popular today is a myth. Simply changing the color tone on your phone screen from blue to yellow puts you in the clear is doing nothing to help you fall asleep at night. It's still light. It's also completely disregarding all the other sources of artificial light besides your devices: overhead lights, bedside lamps, TVs, clock radios, even the sleep and meditation app on your phone that is supposed to help you sleep better. Any source of nighttime light that does not come from nature—such as the moon, stars, planets—will delay how fast you fall asleep. And once you do fall asleep, that exposure will influence your overall quality of sleep. Any exposure to light from any of those things in the hours before you go to bed is impacting your sleep. Nightlights aren't even exempt from this rule! I've treated children for anxiety and depression, only to find out they've been sleeping all night with a nightlight on. We frequently find it much more effective to remove their fear of the dark than to battle against the sleep disruption from having an artificial light on all night.

Another method we use with our sleep study clients is having them wear special glasses with a coating that blocks out ultraviolet light for two hours before bedtime, such as "The Sleep Doctor" Michael Breus's Luminere glasses.[39] This is a very inexpensive strategy that everyone can try; you don't need to be in a sleep study. It's important that you put the glasses on around the same time every night though, in order to retrain your body's circadian rhythm.

The proven relationship between artificial light and sleep problems is also why some psychologists prescribe camping for insomnia and certain mental health disorders. What they're in reality prescribing is circadian rhythm regulation, because when you're camping, you're not exposed to sources of artificial light, and your body will automatically return to a healthy sleep-wake cycle based on the patterns of light and dark in the natural environment—the way we're hard-wired. In addition to helping reset your internal circadian rhythms, studies show that being in nature, and just touching certain kinds of soil, has an antidepressant effect.

We were designed to live in conjunction with our natural world, but we've created a very artificial world that we're now forcing our bodies to adjust to. In the grand scheme of things, we're in the evolutionary phase of a fairly new world where we can live in an artificial environment 24-7, never go outside and rarely have human contact (devices not withstanding) and somehow we still survive. But not thrive, because our bodies aren't designed for this. Our sleep quality and overall health are declining, and daily stress levels are rising as a result of what we consider normal in the new age of technology. Most of our species has entered a state of chronic, acute sleep dysregulation, and the resulting exhaustion is keeps us in a state of overactive stress every day.

Proper Sleep Climate

Light is not the only thing that requires some adjustment for optimal sleep climate. In addition to avoiding artificial light for two hours before bedtime and removing it from your bedroom so it is as dark as possible, you should also adjust the temperature so it's a cool temperature. It's better to have to bundle up a little than to sleep in a warm bedroom.

Next, although they are never great for your stress level, especially avoid content that might trigger stress before bed, such as political talking heads, crime scene investigations, documentaries about serial killers... those images and ideas will creep into your dreams. Even exercise, which is normally a fantastic stress reducer, can be an activator by raising cortisol too close to bedtime. And stimulants such as caffeine are, well, stimulants, so they will prompt your nervous system in the wrong direction as well.

If removing artificial light and altering a person's sleep space and habits isn't enough to restore a patient's circadian rhythms, the root cause of their sleep problems may be more severe. We can add supplements, TouchPoints, and other targeted neural regulation therapies to reset their brain's sleep patterns. There are also certain, more serious problems with sleep that are outside of the scope of this book, and for those I recommend a sleep specialist.

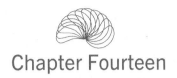

Chapter Fourteen

LIVE WIRES

Post-traumatic stress disorder (PTSD) creates frayed, exposed live wires that are very touchy inside of the nervous system, and that's why PTSD can trigger the stress switch so often and without warning. Live wires are open for triggering the brain's sympathetic response, and in PTSD they've become too sensitive and can spark uncontrollably. What do electricians do when there are exposed wires? They coat the wires to a state where they're no longer exposed and causing problems.

The War at Home

PTSD is diagnosed after a traumatic experience or series of traumatic experiences occurs and an individual's nervous system is not able to return to its pre-trauma level of regulation for a month or more after the event(s).[40] People with PTSD may experience problems sleeping, disturbing intrusive memories, active avoidance of things that remind them of the trauma, an increased startle response or irritation and anger, anxiety, and depression. Although these symptoms can occur in milder forms when someone experiences excess stress, a person with PTSD will experience most of these symptoms on a regular basis and the symptoms are usually more severe. For the PTSD-affected person, the symptoms are specific to a critical incident or set of incidents, and they cause more chronic, debilitating impairments.

The events that precede PTSD are not necessarily life-or-death events, nor are they isolated to experiences of war, car accidents, childhood trauma, or near-death experiences. Many doctors diagnose PTSD only if someone has experienced death, serious injury, sexual violation, or the threat of any of those. However, I've seen PTSD occur from the threat of a relationship loss and other causes that leave many people, especially women, undiagnosed.

Valerie

Valerie was married to a man with a personality disorder, which allowed him to function on a daily basis, but made it hard for him to sustain healthy relationships. As a result of his disorder, Valerie's husband engaged in a high level of constant manipulation, downloaded his work stresses onto her daily, and created a lot of drama and stress, which constantly engulfed his wife's sunny disposition like thunderstorm clouds.

Eventually, she could no longer distinguish the clouds from the horizon, and therefore didn't see the storm she was in the middle of every day. She stayed busy scrambling to keep things together in her life, righting one piece of patio furniture in the backyard at a time, only to have the storm come through and blow everything over again. She simply wasn't able to see how his personality and the dynamics of their marriage turned on her stress switch to an extreme degree of fight-or-flight. Over time, she entered a chronic state of excess stress.

Attempts at couple's therapy resulted in him storming out of the room in a defensive rage, leaving Valerie in tears. He lashed out at her with personal attacks whenever she tried to have a productive conversation about their marriage, and Valerie felt very helpless from not knowing what to do. While her husband had an ACEs score of nine, Valerie had a very low ACEs score, and therefore she was unaccustomed to the pattern of chronic stress that her husband had been living with for most of his life. He was used to constant turmoil, whereas she recognized it as something that needed to be fixed but was powerless to do so.

For Valerie, being under constant low-grade stress gave way to what we call a period of vulnerability. When someone's stress switch is chronically activated into higher levels due to a situation like Valerie's or a pre-existing medical or psychological issue, an extremely upsetting event doesn't have to be life-threatening in order to turn their world upside-down and result in PTSD.

For Valerie, finding out that her husband was having an emotional affair with a co-worker was the PTSD-triggering incident. Some experts disagree that non-life-threatening events such as this could trigger outright PTSD. But I would point out to them that the period of vulnerability beforehand was a compounding factor which raised Valerie's susceptibility to having her stress switch quickly turned from her chronic state of merely "activated" to a high setting. A good analogy would be that when you are sleep-deprived, not exercising, and eating poorly, your immune system is weakened, and you are more susceptible to the flu if you are exposed to it.

Some people might dismiss the severity of Valerie's trauma by saying, "Well, if it wasn't a physical affair, it wasn't really an affair." But studies show that an emotional affair can be just as devastating as a physical affair. In Valerie's case, she had learned of the affair before it became physical. But in doing so, she also learned that her husband had indeed planned on escalating the affair to a physical level at his next opportunity.

Finding out about her husband's emotional affair rocked Valerie's sense of safety because, as difficult as he was, he was a source of security for her. She'd always thought, "Well, at least he's honest and faithful." Without that belief as a security blanket to protect her, she went into an emotional tailspin of stress, fear, and poor sleep; and the resulting cognitive distortions led to her become obsessed with learning everything she could about her husband's affair partner.

What finally brought Valerie into treatment were not the years of constant low-grade stress stemming from her husband's personality disorder. It wasn't even the trauma and shock of her husband's affair. No, Valerie finally sought treatment because her unstable husband, citing the cognitive and systemic symptoms of Valerie's chronic fight-or-flight activation, accused her of having borderline personality disorder. Continuing his pattern of manipulation, he used her symptoms to try to make the case that she was "crazy."

Valerie was not "crazy" at all. She was suffering from PTSD caused by a period of chronic stress activation, followed by a significant event that rocked her sense of safety and security. And statistically, she is not a rare case.

I see children in my office whose parents have habitually exposed them to violent content on the news each night, putting them in a state of chronic low-grade stress, and then when the child personally experiences violence, like watching one of their friends get beat up, it triggers PTSD.

After a lightning bolt struck a flagpole at my children's school, one of their classmates came to my clinic with signs of an acute stress response. As it turned out, the child had been watching content on YouTube about people dying or nearly dying from lightning strikes. He didn't even see the lightning strike the flagpole—which also did not actually strike any person—he'd just watched videos of people talking about what it was like to be struck by lightning. His feelings of vulnerability and thinking about the possibility of death could have easily developed this child's acute stress response into PTSD, had his parents not brought him in for treatment. Fortunately, it did not because we were able to undo the effects in a few EMDR therapy sessions and TouchPoints use at home daily for a few weeks.

These two stories show in vivid detail why I compare a nervous system in PTSD to exposed electrical wires. Once stress exposes the wire, it has the capacity to be sparked out-of-control in an instant by new stressors.

Live Wires

Just like a live electric wire, a constantly and overly triggered nervous system can short-circuit the object it's attached to as well as cause damage to anything else in its path. When water hits exposed wires in a house, the whole house is affected. Just like that, when one person has unchecked excess stress, everyone around that person is affected, and when those people merge into groups, whole communities and entire societies can develop overactive stress switches.

Exposed live wires are a danger to anything around them, and that's what the raw, unpredictably triggered state of PTSD is like. The person moves erratically in and out of fight-or-flight mode, exhibiting all the effects we've talked about in this section—avoidance, selfishness, insomnia, cognitive issues, and more—but in PTSD, the symptoms are at extreme, sometimes dangerous levels. As a result, PTSD doesn't just damage the person's life, relationships, and career. In many cases, it ruins those things. Live wires spark fires.

How PTSD Works

A tripwire is an extremely delicate thread or wire set to operate an explosive alarm or reaction when it is disturbed. Where the (at least moderately adjustable) stress switch used to be, PTSD sets up new, dangerously sensitive tripwires in the neural circuitry of the brain. Normally, when you experience something upsetting or traumatic, your fear and memory systems work in conjunction, adjusting your stress switch up or down to activate your sympathetic nervous system appropriately and dictate behavior that will save your life. In PTSD, the protective and moderating mechanisms in the individual's nervous system are damaged or destroyed, similar to the way insulated coating on electric wires is worn or stripped away, leaving them fragile and exposed. Thus damaged, the PTSD-affected nervous system is full of exposed tripwires that produce a pattern of constantly triggered extreme reactivity that can progress to the point of ruining the person's life.

So instead of getting too close to a drop-off on a hike, sliding a little, and then avoiding that particular spot in the future, with PTSD, the brain memorizes all the sights and sounds of the experience, groups them together under the category of "danger," and sets tripwires to go off in response to any *one* of those factors—a hot sunny day, the smell of pine needles, or the sound of dirt crunching under your hiking boots. Experiencing any of these things could potentially set off a cascade of fight-or-flight responses, and the obsessive thinking characteristic of post-traumatic stress disorder kicks in and you find yourself worrying, "Will going out for a walk on a sunny day kill me?"

Jean

PTSD triggers don't have expiration dates, either. They often increase in sensitivity over time. I had a sixty-five year-old patient named Jean who was sexually abused as a child. Jean didn't fully remember some of the trauma, yet still ended up coping with the results her entire life. At one point, a male co-worker had moved into the cubicle beside her and even though Jean couldn't put her finger on why, he had disgusted her. She had gone to great lengths to avoid him, and even began calling in sick to avoid being around him. She told me she thought she must be going crazy, since this poor man had never actually done anything to her! Meanwhile, her stress level was suddenly through the roof; she was having vague nightmares about her childhood, and flashbacks of memories with hazy outlines. This previously contented woman was now living in an emotional hell, and the worst part was, she had no idea why.

Come to find out, Jean's new co-worker wore Old Spice cologne, just like her abusive father had done, and that sole sensory trigger set off a PTSD cascade. The Old Spice was sensory information, processed in the salience network, which set off her fight-or-flight response — sixty-five years later.

It didn't matter that Jean couldn't consciously recall all the details of the abuse. The frayed, hyper-sensitive livewires activated latent reactivity that had always been there waiting for circumstances that would trigger her stress switch into a pattern of fight-or-flight.

PTSD ID

Many people with PTSD see themselves as permanently damaged goods. This is because of the mood congruent memory concept we discussed in Chapter 8: our memories are colored by our mood. But just like many of the other symptoms of overactive stress, mood congruent memory issues also become more pronounced, even extreme, for people with PTSD, so that they may be unable to access memories colored by happiness. Even if they have a vague awareness of those memories, they don't see a path back to those emotions. They firmly believe that their current state of depression, anger, and anxiety, is permanent.

People with PTSD can begin to own their potentially temporary condition as a part of their permanent identity. They may say, "I'm a just another vet with PTSD," as though this is what their life will be forever, and they have no choice in the matter. Unfortunately, well-meaning doctors and society reinforce this idea of permanency, but it doesn't need to be there.

Addiction and PTSD

Anything that is rewarding and that regulates you can become a behavioral addiction. Because people with PTSD have a higher need for regulation, potentially any substance or behavior that is rewarding is *extra* rewarding to their over-stressed brain—and thus more likely to lead to addiction. I'm talking here about shopping, gambling, drinking alcohol, eating frosting by the spoonful, smoking, obsessively checking Tinder...anything. Studies have shown that when you're stressed, you're more likely to become addicted or relapse with addictive behavior that was previously under control.[41]

People with PTSD are more susceptible to addiction because their stress switches are more easily and frequently activated, and the need for behaviors that dim it down—regardless of long-term consequences—is increased. They are particularly at risk for addiction during the vulnerable time period between when they first develop PTSD symptoms and when they seek treatment.

This is one of many reasons that PTSD should be seen as an urgent, traumatic condition requiring immediate treatment. And by treatment, it should come as no surprise that I don't mean teaching someone how to "cope" with PTSD—I mean getting rid of it, eliminating all excess nervous system reactivity above and beyond what is considered normal. I mean treatment that brings the individual back to a regulated state, restores their pre-PTSD emotional baseline—and in some cases, improves it—and returns their addiction potential to its pre-PTSD baseline. This kind of outcome is not only possible, but in fact it exists today, in the form of EMDR, neurofeedback, and the other therapies we use at the Serin Center clinics and which are available elsewhere as well.

Urgent Care

PTSD is an urgent condition requiring expedient care. Adopting the notion that what doesn't kill you makes you stronger and waiting to treat it can be a deadly. Frequent and extreme nervous system hyper-reactivity wreaks havoc on an individual's life. Resiliency is not built through repeated episodes of damage and repair; it can only come through expedient treatment and proper recovery. We need to start thinking about sympathetic hyper-reactivity and PTSD as conditions necessitating urgent care. We wouldn't let a gaping, infected wound fester, and not go to the doctor right away. Yet we don't see the symptoms of acute stress following traumatic events as requiring the same kind of urgent care.

What does an electrician do when there are exposed wires in someone's home? They coat the wires immediately to prevent the residents from being harmed. What does the medical system typically do when those exposed live wires are in a human being with a life, relationships, career, goals, and dreams?

Well, I will say that they have the chemical aspect of the solution well covered, offering trauma patients drugs that mute the nervous system's reactions in hopes of warding off PTSD. These drugs lower the physiological reactivity of the sympathetic nervous system, and in doing so, they disrupt the way the fear and memory networks link up so they can't work together to create those exposed live wires.

However, this search for the perfect chemical cocktail is overcomplicating what PTSD is and how it works. Also, we're often prescribing medications that aren't necessarily recommended by the World Health Organization or other reputable organizations like *Cochrane Reviews*. We're telling people it's a chronic problem, sending them off with prescriptions, including addictive anti-anxiety medications, and telling them nothing else can be done. The result is that people with PTSD are left on their own to calm their hyper-reactive nervous systems with coping strategies like alcohol, street drugs, and bad habits. When those strategies don't calm them down, they succumb to irritability, anger, daggers, lashing out and even violence, leaving a string of broken relationships, lost jobs, and ruined potential in their wake. It doesn't need to be this way.

Treating PTSD

When treating PTSD, a nervous system reset is necessary. In movie production, the phrase "back to one" means the actors and the camera go back to where they were at the beginning of the scene. Effective PTSD treatment brings a person back to where they were, in terms of their nervous system reactivity, prior to the trauma. Treatment that does not accomplish this is not enough. Merely putting Band-Aids on someone's symptoms not only allows the live wires in their nervous system to continue sparking uncontrollably; but the symptoms will become more and more erratic over time, causing more and more damage to everyone and everything around it.

Not only can we achieve a "back to one" scenario after PTSD; we can often do better than that. With treatments such as neurofeedback, EMDR, TouchPoints, and others, we can actually improve someone's baseline functioning beyond what it was before the trauma. Finally, some good news!

We need two things to treat PTSD effectively. Number one, we need to create conditions that reduce the patient's nervous system reactivity during both the day and night. That involves ongoing homeostatic and nervous system regulation, accomplished by treatment modalities like TouchPoints and meditation along with a foundation of healthy behaviors.

Number two, we need to help people with PTSD process the trauma so their stress switches are not so reactive. At the time of this book's writing, the gold standards for this are trauma-focused CBT and EMDR therapy.

No matter how we treat PTSD, the sooner we do it, the better the outcome. One of the barriers to quick treatment is how long before the condition is diagnosed. Before one month elapses after a trauma, similar symptoms are called acute stress disorder, and many say that while EMDR therapy and trauma-focused CBT are appropriate for PTSD, they should not be used to treat acute stress disorder. That's like saying a water hose can be used against a burning house, but not for the kitchen fire that caused it. Ignore the small fire and all you'll have to look forward to is fighting a much bigger, more out-of-control fire. It's that simple.

If Valerie had sought treatment for the stress symptoms caused by her chronically stressful marriage before finding out about her husband's affair, the trauma of the affair may not have caused PTSD. We can prevent PTSD, and we also can treat it right away once it happens. It does not have to be a disorder that ruins people's lives, because it's simply a neurological issue resulting from trauma. We can recoat the exposed live wires so that they're not tripwires in the brain anymore, setting off cascades of uncontrollable sympathetic activation. We can help the brain recover. We can give people their lives and full potential back.

Preventing PTSD

In my consulting work with foreign militaries, I have been asked, "How do we make sure that nobody gets PTSD?" The question is so big and important, and I started thinking about whether we could prevent PTSD the same way vaccines prevent viral infections.

Earlier in the book, I mentioned volunteer EMDR therapists who respond to global crises through Trauma Recovery, EMDR Humanitarian Assistance Programs. [42] Trauma Recovery/HAP volunteers have observed that if an entire village experiences systemic trauma like a tsunami, a certain percentage of the group will develop PTSD afterwards. Data collected from their work suggests that if the volunteers can get to the village, treat the individuals with PTSD symptoms fairly quickly, they can essentially eradicate PTSD almost entirely!

For example, in response to the 1999 earthquake in Marmara, Turkey, Trauma Recovery/HAP volunteers trained therapists after the earthquake to conduct five, ninety-minute EMDR sessions with survivors in tents. The result? A 92.7 percent elimination of the PTSD symptoms in the participants treated.[43] And, if a person goes through a devastating earthquake, gets treated, comes out with no PTSD, and the brain now has a pattern of recovering completely after going through devastation, what do you think will happen if another tragedy strikes? The data from Marmara suggests that, unless there is a physical injury or another mitigating circumstance, that person will be less likely to develop PTSD the second time. This looks like the definition of resilience.

These results go against a commonly held belief that when multiple traumatic incidents affect one person, or one population of people, the stress and trauma accumulate. On the contrary, they show that after people are exposed to a traumatic stressor, if they receive the right kind of treatment, and quickly, not only can people recover fully from PTSD, but also that the treatment may also inoculate a certain percentage of the population against PTSD caused by future trauma, similar to how vaccines work.

A vaccine contains a small, inactive dose of a virus. While the dose is too small to cause harm, the immune system responds to its presence by teaching itself how to produce antibodies that respond to that particular virus. In this way, if a vaccinated person gets exposed to the active virus later, the body will know how to respond. It will have experience and information gained from being exposed to a low dose of that particular threat in the past.

If a vaccine contained too large a dose, or if the virus were to be active, it would quickly overpower the immune system and disease would wreak havoc on the person's body. This is similar to what we see can happen with PTSD.

When people can obtain immediate treatment after trauma strikes, resiliency builds. In a sense, they are building up immunity to stress—with a "low dose" of traumatic activation—against a more serious future case of PTSD. But in other cases, where the individuals do not receive speedy treatment before their symptoms progress to damaging levels, they receive too high a "dose" of active stress, and their bodies react with full-blown disease rather than developing resiliency.

This is why correct and fast treatment is vital, like the EMDR therapy HAP volunteers administered to the villagers. EMDR is just one example of a "right" treatment; my emphasis here is on speed of treatment. An urgent approach can cut down immensely the number of people who will develop full-blown PTSD after being exposed to large stressors like abuse, a life-threatening illness or injury, or war. If and we're treating the symptoms of acute stress right away rather than simply muting and masking the symptoms, and as a result we're dealing with a smaller number of PTSD cases, I believe we can eradicate it just as we've eradicated the global threat of diseases like polio over the years.

Diseases like polio still exist in the world, albeit on an incredibly small scale compared to where they once were. I went to a hotel once where the lobby was decorated with vintage signs and artifacts. One of the signs was a public reminder from the early 20th century for people to wash their hands to prevent polio. Polio was on everybody's minds then because it could create highly destructive physical and neurological outcomes for people. I think it's safe to say that polio is no longer top-of-mind for people in terms of the things we worry about on a daily basis. But this isn't to say we're entirely safe from it.

The backlash against vaccines, largely based on the erroneous and scientifically unproven notion that they cause autism, could open the door for the resurgence of polio, smallpox, measles, and other devastating diseases. These diseases still very much exist; they have by no means been cured, and they can come back if we allow it.

Think about how quickly medical science progresses. Just seventy years ago, polio was on everyone's mind, and we've basically conquered it. Now, PTSD is one of the diseases that has replaced it as a major problem. But just as the solution to epidemics of polio began with understanding how to create immunity to it, our best treatments may not only halt the progress of PTSD, but also potentially confer immunity for the future. These new treatments and technologies are also giving everybody better access to homeostatic regulation in real time, and improving the way that we respond to and adapt to stressors in our daily lives. We can eliminate people's periods of vulnerability and treat acute stress and PTSD right after exposure to a traumatic stressor, bring them back to homeostatic regulation, and repair the neural circuitry of their brains.

But instead, the majority of PTSD patients are being told to cope with their condition. Coping with PTSD means taking your anti-anxiety meds, meditating, and sending your partner to support networks to talk about what it's like to live with somebody with PTSD. They're taught how to manage the situation, how to be empathetic, how to shield themselves, and how to call 911 if they feel like their life is in danger. These should be temporary strategies at best, employed only while the individual's care team is actively working to fix the problem of a constantly overstimulated nervous system. It's not a good use of anyone's time to spend twenty hours training a partner on how to live with live wires that can essentially set the whole house on fire.

This applies to any type of acute stress disorder or stress-triggered neurological reactivity, not just PTSD. I saw a child almost get expelled for throwing chairs in class and yelling at his teacher. He was regularly launching into full-blown flight-or-flight, and acting like an animal. This boy did not necessarily have PTSD. He had something called intermittent explosive disorder, which is another variation of a triggered sympathetic nervous system.

The school tried to help the parents cope with their child's out-of-control behavior. They actually sat down with the boy and tried to talk his stress switch into turning off, creating strategies for him to "think before he acts." None of this addressed the actual nervous system problem. The live wire was bouncing around the floor, throwing sparks everywhere, and everyone was dancing around it and running for cover, but not calling an electrician to do something about it.

This avoidance wreaked havoc on the family's life as they moved from school to school, leaving a wake of ruined relationships. On top of that, the child felt so bad, especially right after the incidents, tearfully telling his parents, "I don't know what got into me." Well, when they brought him to me, I knew. It was plain to see that his fight-or-flight system was intermittently taking over his body and as we know, he was helpless to do anything about it.

Aside from teachers who don't have the medical training to know better, there are many well-meaning practitioners in the PTSD space who are still ignoring the mercury in the pond, cleaning off one rock at a time, one symptom at a time, with a toothbrush. They're inventing expensive, overcomplicated, albeit creative, ways to help people calm down their PTSD symptoms while they're in treatment. Then the person goes home, is left to rely on personal coping skills, cognitive or self-help strategies, and when those fail, the person is right back where they started, battling the internal live wires of an overstimulated nervous system. These are all beautiful efforts by people who truly care, but they are not fixing the problem. Unless we do the right things at the right time to repair how the nervous system functions, we're really just putting a Band-Aid over a bullet wound—or duct tape over a sparking live wire.

If more people understood all this, PTSD would not be a multi-billion dollar problem that is ruining lives. If we approached PTSD as the neurological, fluctuating nervous system problem it is, I believe we could wipe out perhaps 80-90 percent of it globally. I would like to see that happen in my lifetime.

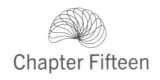

Chapter Fifteen

AFTER THE BREAKDOWN

Given what you learned in the first part of this book about how your nervous system works and what you've seen in this second part about the serious consequences of excess stress run amok, can you see that just coping with it makes absolutely no sense? When your stress switch is set on high, trying to talk yourself into coping strategies is impossible because your body is trying to survive; it doesn't particularly care that you're trying to have a conversation about "calming down." Coping requires planning, conscious thinking, and organizing what you're going to do in response to certain situations. How can you do that when you're in fight-or-flight? You can't. When your stress switch is cranked beyond a low setting, you need more powerful tools than what your mind alone can provide.

I hope I've also convinced you that even if self-talk, planning, and even drugs *were* effective coping strategies for stress, "coping" itself is settling for far less than what is available—because there are treatments that can often eliminate the excess stress and its symptoms altogether. Telling someone to cope with excess stress is telling them to find a way to function well in a state of constant reactivity and manage all its effects, from performance issues and selfishness, to more serious issues such as sleep disorders and the lives wires of PTSD. Managing these symptoms requires immense effort and takes away from a happy, healthy, and fulfilling life. It is exhausting, expensive, and time-consuming.

People who have struggled with addiction understand this well, because even when they're sober they are still forced to cope with irritability, cravings, withdrawal symptoms, insomnia, and more. A lot of energy goes into not using a substance. Now, if we change their brain so that they will crave the substance less and less, or so they'll react to it less, the amount of time and effort that they'll need to invest into resisting the behavior goes down exponentially. And then, they can get truly get their lives back.

In the same way, we can change the brain for people struggling to manage out-of-control stress, to give them a fighting chance to conquer the beast once and for all. This is my goal in the treatment of stress—to help people suffering from it to get their lives back. I won't quit until we completely get rid of the all these problems (and more) reactivity has caused for individuals, their communities, and our entire world.

Our societal habit of accepting mere coping strategies is a big obstacle to this change. But now that you know that the stress situation is more changeable than you thought, we can embark on the final conversation of this book, about what it takes to really move on.

Now, even if you are a very high-functioning person who is not experiencing the majority of topics covered in this past section of the book, it's important to realize that your nervous system is fluctuating just like anybody else's. Whether you are aware of dealing with external stressors or not, you are still susceptible to past thoughts and situations triggering your stress switch from peaceful to stressed out mode. Maybe your switch is moving microscopically, just enough to throw you off-balance, take you out of your optimal zone of high performance, focus, and clear, critical thinking—all the things that will give you access to your highest human potential. Even mild activation can ruin performance.

No one is immune to micro-triggers that move the stress switch. Even experienced meditators experience stress that registers on the stress switch scale—they just experience a smaller increase than the rest of us. Just like the Olympic athletes who can hold their breath longer, through intense training they've increased their body's capacity. This is very good for those lucky few who can dedicate so much of their life to skill-building like that. And not so good for the rest of us who've sat on a mat and tried to meditate, only to become frustrated and feel like a failure when we "can't get into the zone." For the rest of us there are TouchPoints—and this book, which is a user's manual for your nervous system.

Take a moment to explore the how your stress switch may be specifically affecting you personally—even to a small degree. Think about the whole spectrum, from mild to severe, in all the categories we've discussed: emotions, focus, productivity, performance, sleep, intimacy, relationships, communication, and health.

If you have trouble identifying areas where your stress switch flipping on is even a mild factor in your life, close your eyes for a moment and picture the last time you were stressed or simply out-of-balance: running late, irritated by something or someone, working on insufficient sleep, confronting a conversation you wanted to avoid, or in general not having a great day. We all have at least one thing about our lives that triggers us, and therefore triggers our stress switch.

Yes, we can do things like meditate for temporary relief. But wouldn't it be ideal to remove the nervous system activation around those triggers, for good? You can take your discovery to the next level by asking these questions: what parts of your life do you wish weren't a part of your life? If a magic genie could deal with certain people in your life or resolve certain situations outright for you, what would you wish for?

Now imagine this on a national or even global level. Our entire species eradicating this plague called stress, one trigger at a time. In learning to treat ourselves, we'll no longer be contributing to the epidemic of stress. We'll also be nurturing what's best about ourselves. The new world of human beings realizing our full potential begins when our ancient, intelligently designed but dumb nervous systems are no longer getting in our way.

Part III: Victory

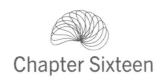

Chapter Sixteen

FLIP YOUR OWN SWITCH FIRST

A series of *Snickers* chocolate bar commercials remind us, "You're not you when you're hungry." Well, as you just saw in Part II, you're not you when you're stressed, either. When you're stressed, you're selfish, combative, sleep-deprived, and you perform badly; your reality becomes cognitively distorted with lies made up by your triggered mind as you relive past traumas and make negative predictions about the future... and the list goes on. Your whole person is compromised. The most urgent order of business for you is to flip your own stress switch off and get the real you back online again.

Flight attendants on airplanes tell us to put our own oxygen masks on first, and then put them on children or others needing assistance. It's become almost a cliché, yet it's true of so many other things in life that, order to help others, we must tend to ourselves first. In order to "be the change we wish to see in the world," we must operate from a calm nervous system as much as possible, with our stress switch in the off position.

So first, you deal with your own stress switch. Think of your first goal as establishing a new, baseline for the calmest, healthiest life humanly possible. Only then can you begin to deal with other people's contagious stress switches. Besides minimizing the problems of one compromised person trying to "fix" another one, there's another reason to start with yourself. If you don't deal with your own stress first, not only will you be a ball of reactivity, likely to perpetuate the other person's stress instead of really helping, you'll also be seeing others through the fog and cognitive distortions of fight-of-flight, and therefore you won't accurately see their needs.

Knowledge is power, and if the first level of empowerment is being aware of and managing your own stress switch, the second level is to set an example for others and educate them about how stress works. You now have an advantage, since you are a person who understands stress in the human body and how the stress switch works. You can now look at situations around you, whether involving your significant other, your children, other family members, friends, coworkers, or even strangers in public, and realize that when someone "goes off," in all likelihood they are not some sort of psychopath. You will know that for whatever reason, their stress switch has been flipped and they are lost in the physical effects of fight-or-flight. Armed with the knowledge from this book, you will be able to risk the contagion of their stress and respond more helpfully.

Finally comes the highest level of knowledge empowerment of all—being a part of the paradigm shift itself. Throughout this book I have laid out my vision for shifting the current paradigm of coping with stress to a new paradigm of curing the public health epidemic that stress really is. Armed with new awareness and knowledge, you are now in a position to help me realize that vision. I invite you to take the understanding that stress is not something in your head that you must outwit, but rather a physical condition in the body that can be switched off, and put that knowledge to good use.

In this final section of the book, we will look at all three levels of the empowerment hierarchy: taking control of your own stress switch, creating awareness in others around you, and then working together to turn off the global stress switch.

There are certain foundational behaviors that affect your daily stress levels and therefore your baseline. One thing I'm *not* going to do here is attempt to write a specific prescription for all the actions you need to take in each area of your life to reduce your stress. The idea is to move away from the stress-producing expectation that you have to do fifty things perfectly in order to have a great life. Stress management itself becomes stressful when you are told that you need to eat a certain ratio of protein to carbohydrates to fats every three to four hours a day, do twenty minutes of cardio and ten minutes of weightlifting, and thirty minutes of meditation every morning, and go to yoga on Thursdays.

Rather than going that route, I've created an assessment you can use to identify and rank potential sources of stress in your life based on how easy they would be to change. My goal is to show you that taking action—even small actions—is a doable method of lowering your stress and then maintaining a calm baseline for your life. You might not necessarily keep your stress switch in the totally off position right away; but if you can lower it from where it is now, that's a victory.

For the following assessment, I recommend using a journal or notebook to consider each of the questions from several perspectives. First, consider, "Is this true in my life?" Then, follow up by asking, "How easy would this be to change?" Use "0" to indicate "easiest" and "10" for "hardest." Finally, make a note of the steps you think you will need to change the behavior. For example, for sleep, the steps might be to 1) set an alarm on your cell phone to alert you when it's bedtime; 2) prioritize sleep over watching a show or checking social media; 3) block off bedtime on your calendar so you don't schedule social events too late at night, 4) set a reminder to go to bed early when you need to wake up early the next day, etc. Once you've considered all the questions, your goal will be to go back and rank the areas *against each other*, not just against your overall resistance.

In your current situation and based on the last three months of your life:

1. Do you get 7-9 hours of sleep most nights?

How easy would this be to change?
(0 = easy, 10 = hard)

List the steps you'd be willing to try if you aren't getting enough sleep.

How does this rank relative to the other areas?
(1 = easiest, 9 = hardest)

2. Do you gossip or spend a lot of time in conversations complaining?

How easy would this be to change?
(0 = easy, 10 = hard)

List the steps you'd be willing to try to change this behavior if you engage in gossip about others or complain.

How does this rank relative to the other areas?
(1 = easiest, 9 = hardest)

3. Do you hold onto anger when you've been wronged?

How easy would this be to change?
(0 = easy, 10 = hard)

List steps you'd be willing to try to let go of anger if anger hijacks your calm states.

How does this rank relative to the other areas?
(1 = easiest, 9 = hardest)

4. Do you get and stay upset about things beyond your control like politics or other people's behavior?

How easy would this be to change?
(0 = easy, 10 = hard)

List the steps you'd be willing to try to ease up on the upset if you stay upset about things outside of your control.

How does this rank relative to the other areas?
(1 = easiest, 9 = hardest)

5. **Do you invest excessive time in thinking about a person (or people) who bothers you?**

How easy would this be to change?
(0 = easy, 10 = hard)

List the steps you'd be willing to try to stop obsessing about others if you can't seem to shut this out of your mind.

How does this rank relative to the other areas?
(1 = easiest, 9 = hardest)

6. **Do you feel like you spend excessive time being pessimistic or making negative predictions?**

How easy would this be to change?
(0 = easy, 10 = hard)

List the steps you'd be willing to try to become more of a positive thinker if your negativity often weighs you down.

How does this rank relative to the other areas?
(1 = easiest, 9 = hardest)

7. **Do you have a healthy go-to way of coping or eliminating with sudden bouts of stress (TouchPoints, breathing exercises, meditation, exercise, a support network of friends, an outside professional like a therapist or counselor you can call, religious or spiritual practices, etc.)?**

How easy would this be to change?
(0 = easy, 10 = hard)

List the steps you'll need to create healthy go-to behaviors if you don't have healthy ways of coping with or eliminating stress in the moment.

How does this rank relative to the other areas?
(1 = easiest, 9 = hardest)

8. **Do you have a set of daily habits designed to keep your stress switch off and your calm baseline low (Yoga, meditation, journaling, writing in a gratitude journal, exercise, TouchPoints, etc.)?**

How easy would this be to change?
(0 = easy, 10 = hard)

List the steps you'll need to establish a set of daily habits and rank order which ones might be the most important for you to start or modify.

How does this rank relative to the other areas?
(1 = easiest, 9 = hardest)

9. **Do you have a social network of supportive friends, family members, professional helpers, or others who you can turn to when you are upset or when life events are difficult?**

How easy would this be to change?
(0 = easy, 10 = hard)

List the steps you'll need to cultivate a support network if you feel like you don't have one established.

How does this rank relative to the other areas?
(1 = easiest, 9 = hardest)

Now, rank all the actions in order from 1-9, starting with the "easiest to change" behavior at "1", all the way up to behaviors that may need more work over the longer term. Easy behaviors may take little effort or time to change and feel less like impossible-to-break habits. No ties are allowed. This will help you clearly see the best place to start so you can start benefitting from better habits as soon as possible. Ranking also replaces the idea that some behaviors are impossible to change with the much more constructive reality that it some things just take a little longer or require more energy and effort.

Everything you do expends energy and has an opportunity cost. When you invest energy and effort into one activity, it takes away from something else you could be doing. This is why the time investment of stress management often stresses people out.

Modifying the easiest-to-change behaviors first will give you the momentum and positive reinforcement to keep working your way up to the more challenging ones. Start small and work your way up. Take a bite out of the stress management elephant rather than attempting to swallow it whole. Every positive action you take toward lowering your stress switch in your daily life will lower your calm baseline, keep you out of fight-or-flight more and more, and turn what you once considered to be inevitable, possibly even chronic, stress into isolated, rare, and fixable events.

Your goal is to create enough positive habits to keep your stress switch off as much as possible. That will make your life, and the lives of those around you, ultimately better.

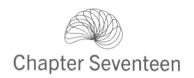

Chapter Seventeen

COLLUSION

Gross! The swimming pool at the Airbnb my family had just checked into had debris bobbing all over the surface, and the water was as green as the Wicked Witch herself in the *Wizard of Oz*.

Since we were going to be there for nine days, in the midst of selling our old home and moving into the new one, I told the property's manager that this would not do, especially with two bored, overheating boys in the middle of an Arizona summer.

First he blamed the storm, but I pointed out that the problem wasn't just leaves and other normal storm debris floating around; the water was *green*! Next, he arrived and tried to clean the pool's pump (something my dad had come by and already tried to do with no success), and when that didn't work, he then accused me of either turning the pump off before he got there or allowing one of the children's toys to jam it (neither of which was true).

At that point my stress switch started to overheat about how unfairly I was being treated by this man. We cleaned his pool ourselves for hours and hours. On top of that, we fixed a fence that blew over in the storm, and when a roof started leaking, we cleaned up the mess and then let him know about it.

Although as far as I knew, we'd been nothing but model guests, when we checked out, this very upset man decided to, from my point of view, declare war on me. He turned into a kind of paparazzi, snapping pictures all over the house showcasing dust and dirt that was there before we'd arrived, and even a Band-Aid on the floor behind a trash can that we'd never moved.

Here I was in the middle of a real estate transaction and a stressful move; it was the hottest week of the summer with temperatures around 116 degrees until the daily monsoon drenched whatever we were doing, and this Airbnb guy was now trying to scam me out of money to clean messes that I didn't cause!

At that point all I could think was: "This is a terrible Airbnb, and I'm ready to let the whole world know about it!" In retrospect, this is *exactly* how many scathing online reviews are born (something I did not do by the way), ones that can do serious damage to a business, all because a consumer gets lost in the heat of the moment with their stress switch on. This, of course, was classic fight-or-flight thinking triggered by situational stress. My stress switch was in the on position; and because of my activated nervous system I was only able to see the worst in that man and the worst of the situation.

And then suddenly, I had a better explanation for his behavior. Unbeknownst to me, during our stay, my son had decided to sneak a protein bar to bed with him in the middle of the night. At the end of our stay, when I tossed our bedding into the washer and dryer, the gooey, food-caked protein bar wrapper was hidden deep in the sheets. As if things weren't already tense enough, the sheets were ruined. The landlord sent me a photo of the messed up sheets and the incriminating wrapper, and angrily informed me that the bill to replace his 1,400-thread count sheets would not be a small one.

I looked at that photo and I had no choice but to acknowledge that I was responsible for the situation. It was my kid's protein bar that destroyed this man's sheets, clear and simple. He wasn't making it up.

Once I zoomed out from my stressed out tunnel vision, I saw the situation clearly. This guy wasn't a professional scam artist, out to rip off innocent Airbnb customers. Like me, he was operating out of fight-or-flight.

This is how wars break out, whether in our lives or on a larger scale. Byron Katie, who is famous for her method of self-inquiry called "The Work," says that war begins with defensiveness. In my initial stressed out state, I started creating all kinds of stories about how this Airbnb guy was trying to scam me. But the honest truth of it was that he was also dealing with the same unrelenting 116-degree heat and daily monsoons, and now he was coming home to a green pool, broken pool pump, and ruined sheets. He was upset, just like anyone else would be, and the totality of the situation set him off. With the cognitive distortion of confirmation bias in full effect one will almost always find the conclusion they're seeking. Therefore, he began seeing other problems around the place, which he naturally aimed the in my direction. He was irrational, but that didn't mean he was "doing anything" to me. I consciously decided that I didn't want to spend any more of my time on the situation; that my life was more important than that temporary drama.

Later that night after my stress switch was finally off, I realized that this was just one blip on the radar of my life and I probably wouldn't even remember it in a year. I knew that hashing and rehashing the situation while in an activated state was not productive for my life. I had hurt myself beyond the situation in making these assumptions about this man whom I barely knew. As soon as I did that, and got out of my defensive "the world is out to get me" victim posture, I felt an emotional release, the incident floated gently behind me into the past, and I moved on.

This situation reinforced a couple of lessons for me. First, I remembered how important it is to constantly be building immunity to the stress around us. Second, I recommitted to stop spending so many moments in a state of upset about stories made up in fight-or-flight. When we open up space and time in our lives to be calm, positive changes will naturally emerge. Then we can keep taking future steps to open up even more of that space to feel calm, better about ourselves, and think about stressful situations with others in a whole new way.

Colluding

A patient tells me, "My wife is trying to make me feel guilty." I tell him, "Actually, she's not." When he looks at me with doubt, I explain that what his wife is doing is setting guilt down on the floor in front of him, and he's choosing to pick it up. It's his choice to collude with the emotions and stress that are part of her emotional state. They do not have to be a part of *his* emotional state unless he takes ownership of them.

My eleven-year-old often says in frustration, "This is too hard, I just can't do this." I'll respond, "Honey, I love you too much to agree with that. I realize you see that as your truth in this moment, but that doesn't mean that you're right." I refuse to collude with the stress that is influencing him to hurt himself by not trying. Women, especially, are taught to be nice and agreeable at all costs, and it's taken me a lifetime to try to break myself of this habit. Sometimes collusion isn't the way to go, and sometimes the agreeable thing isn't the kind thing to do. We use different methods to calm my son's frustration. Fortunately, as I have alluded to throughout this book, there are as many ways to get out of the state of stress as there are to get into it.

Collusion happens frequently in the workplace. Almost every CEO I work with on performance enhancement has the habit of creating time pressure. They self-impose impossible deadlines while gripping tightly to the idea that in order to be right, things must be done a particular way. They believe that if they pressure people and create an atmosphere of stress, things will get done better and faster. In most situations, they set goals using a method I like to call MSU (make something up). This strategy almost always backfires, leading to burnout for the leaders and their employees, with everybody involved feeling like they're never getting enough done and never doing a good enough job.

These teams end up feeling like it's their sole job to bend to the CEO's will, when in reality all they are doing is colluding with the CEO's self-perpetuated stress. My cousin, an engineer, recently shared that his company is under arbitrary deadlines and often produces sub-optimal products as a result. The fallout? Employee burnout and millions of lost dollars on the back-end trying to fix defective products. If we could remove the CEO's chronic stress, the entire cycle could be broken. It often starts by reframing those made-up goals and the stories the CEO has created around what will happen if they are not met.

There's an old parable about a farmer whose horse runs away, and his neighbor thinks "what terrible luck," while the farmer says, "who knows what's good or bad?" When the horse returns with more horses and the neighbor can't believe his good fortune, the farmer says, "who knows what's good or bad?" Then, the farmer's son breaks his leg training one of the horses and the neighbor thinks, "Oh no!" while the farmer again stays calm. Soon, there's a draft to war and the son is spared because of his broken leg.

The moral of the story is that it can be a mistake to spend so much energy toggling back and forth between our judgments of what we want to happen versus what we don't want to happen, and then colluding with the stress of those judgments, instead of just dealing with what is. Our judgments, in and of themselves, can contribute so much additional stress, on top of the stress of an actual incident. We pile on, "isn't this terrible, isn't this awful, isn't it horrible..." You know what? It's actually not over 'til the fat lady sings. When I catch myself thinking these things, I remind myself that I won't be able to tell until I'm on my deathbed which things ended up being a net positive and which ones were a net negative in my own life. And even then, my own judgments will still be filtered through my own myopic lens and not a reflection of the net effect on a grander scale.

For many of us, making value judgments in the moment, and worse, *before* the moment, takes up a lot of time and keeps us in a constant state of stress, worrying about the unknown. Much of the judgment comes from colluding with each other about what should be stressful and what should not. In every culture there's a consensus about what standards we should use to judge things in our lives. If the majority of people think a certain way then it *must* be that way. Right? Not really.

For instance, if you polled fifty people about whether getting laid-off from work is good or bad, forty-five of them would probably say it's bad. But my twenty-something year-old friend would disagree with that poll, because he just got laid-off recently and he's as happy as a clown. He called me on the phone and told me excitedly, "This is awesome! I got a six-month severance package and guess what? I was going to quit anyway!" He refused to collude with popular opinion about what should be stressful, and went with his own, less stressful judgment instead. He didn't take it personally, either, which could have caused him a lot of unnecessary stress. Even though being laid-off was a great thing for him, because he had six months to look for a new job without any financial strain, people around him tried to stress him out about it: "What if it takes you more than six months to find a job?" they asked. "What will you say in an interview to make sure it doesn't look like you failed at this last position?" "Oh no! You won't be able to keep contributing to your 401K for the next six months and that will be awful, terrible...." You get the picture. Luckily, he was hearty enough to not allow his well-meaning but misguided friends and family activate his stress switch. They laid it down but he refused to pick it up.

How do you want to manifest your own personal stress level? How much will you allow yourself to collude with other people's stress and pick up the emotions they lay down on the ground in front of you? We can each make the individual choice as to how much we're willing to let other people's stress impact us, which stressful beliefs we're willing to buy into, and what we'll do in the presence of stress.

Part of what I hope you'll gain from this book is the ability to recognize when people's stress switches are on and they want yours to be on, too. Developing this awareness can help you fend off vicarious stress and refuse to be triggered. When you feel stressed, you might look to the people around you. If their switches have unconsciously triggered you, then take steps to relieve your own stress. I was out to dinner with my friend Nicole and she was getting increasingly upset while recounting a story about something that happened to her recently on a date. I instantly picked up on her stress and suffering, and being a human being with my own nervous system, I began to get a little activated myself, feeling my breathing getting shallow, my heart speeding up. I found it more and more difficult to concentrate on the conversation as my stress switch started to collude with hers.

Thankfully, knowledge is power, and I had tools. I handed her my set of TouchPoints, and she calmed down as she continued on with her story. On my side of the table, I started breathing more deeply, my heart rate slowed down, and I became more present again.

Even those of us who make our living working with the mind are not immune to its age-old programming. A skill that counselors work on for years is how to stay calm when other people are stressed out. They might be able to create an appearance of calm to help their patients calm down, but often their nervous systems are reacting just the way human nervous systems do until they take conscious steps to reduce their reactivity. This is why compassion fatigue is common amongst therapists and also caregivers. Both categories of people absorb the energy emitted by nervous system stress.

Unless you either move to Mars or sequester yourself on that mountaintop in India to meditate for the rest of your life, you're going to be around stressed out people. The goal is to notice when you are in the presence of stress, so you can consciously avoid colluding with it or allowing it to activate your own stress switch.

The Language of Stress

When you understand your stress switch and how it works, one of the ways you can model that understanding and help people is to adopt a belief system and language that is less judgmental towards others.

A colleague of mine, a neurosurgeon, recently observed a waiting room full of family members who were awaiting news of a loved one undergoing major surgery following a serious accident. From his vantage point, he saw a lack of emotion, stony faces, and blank lifeless gazes. Based on his own set of beliefs, he concluded they weren't concerned enough about their loved one. The more he thought about it, the more upset he got, wondering, "What is the *matter* with these people? Why don't they care that their loved one might die?"

In his mind, he labeled the family as uncaring and callous, and as a result his behaviors toward them naturally reflected this judgment, creating an invisible barrier between them. How many times have you done this in life? Made a snap judgment about what someone must be thinking or feeling based on their outer appearance and behaviors?

But the fact was, they were not uncaring at all. They were in "freeze mode"—another typical effect of fight-or-flight. Their bodies were so physically overwhelmed with the chemicals of stress that they completely shut down. The disconnection created by his misjudgment was the exact opposite of what would have been most helpful to calm those worried people.

More understanding and awareness of the stress response can also help when stress makes you behave badly toward someone. When you realize it afterwards, rather than pretending the incident never happened, a more self-aware and empowered choice is to acknowledge the stress elephant in the room, and explain what happened. This also offers an opportunity to explain to someone else how stress works.

Here's how such an apology might sound: "You know what? I'm really sorry I wasn't paying attention to you this morning when you needed me. I was behaving selfishly and defensively. When you were trying to talk to me, I was actually stressed myself, which put my brain in a certain state called fight-or-flight mode that made me want to leave the situation. That is why I wasn't able to pay attention to you and I seemed distant. This is no excuse for my behavior, but I wanted to explain to you what happened so you know it had nothing to do with you or what you were saying to me. I was stressed, but now I've handled that and I'm no longer in that state. I would really like to talk to you now. Would you be willing to do that with me?"

Using this type of language not only helps you understand and take ownership of your own stress, but also helps you move forward in your relationships, avoiding any lingering baggage hanging overhead.

Stripping Away Stress

I don't need to be at Thanksgiving dinner with my patient whose in-laws nitpick her shortcomings in front of everybody to help her with that situation. I can walk her through remembering it and she'll feel similarly to how she felt in the moment.

Put in very simple terms, on a brain scan, her brain activity would functionally change while she remembered the event, similarly as it did in the moment (if someone happened to do a brain scan on her at the Thanksgiving dinner table). This is good news and bad news.

It means we can fix things when we're not in the moment. But it also means we can wreak havoc on ourselves when we're not in the moment, with all these stories that we're telling ourselves. Part of reaching your potential is shortening the duration of time that you're spending in the latter moments, telling yourself these negative prediction stories that that tax your energy and your reserves, or staying preoccupied with a situation that happened before and isn't happening now. These neural habits keep your stress switch on. That's the price we pay for consciousness and, although I wouldn't trade it, it can be a double-edged sword.

How much can we reduce this realistically in life, and then what does that leave room for? Spoiler alert, it leaves room for some amazing things! Because at our core as human beings, when we transcend stress, all that's left is beauty, love, light, joy, and empathy. When people reduce their stress, wonderful things emerge and become possible—enjoying yourself, being productive, connecting with others in meaningful ways, practicing gratitude, and taking actions that benefit others. Those things are all at our core, under all the stress that we're carrying around with us every day in varying levels.

Despite what some would say, I don't think that inner light is lost in most people. I believe the light from one person can change the whole world if it gets bright enough. But stress, especially the chronic daily stress that we actively feed by directing energy toward unnecessary thoughts, dims that light. This is an individual and a global tragedy. Until we fix it.

Behavioral Control

The CEO of PepsiCo, Indra Nooyi, was recounting advice she'd gotten from Steve Jobs. He told her not to be too nice, and if she isn't getting what she believes is the right thing for the company, he said, "it's okay to throw a temper tantrum and throw things around."[44] At Apple, Jobs had a reputation for being condescending and harsh but incredibly productive, and he inspired great loyalty in some employees.

Now, I love Apple products and do not mean to undermine Steve Jobs' brilliance or what he was able to accomplish in his lifetime, but that's terrible advice for most of us. There are many ways to let people know that you're serious. If you're yelling, all they can hear is your anger, which puts them in a state of fight-or-flight. This may lead to temporary compliance, as the adrenaline triggered by the sympathetic reaction keeps them up and working all night to get the job done. I'm not sure that's a managerial win in the long run when all you have are burnt-out people who are no longer able to get any job done, even if you yell. Adrenaline can only take you so far. And while it's true Apple has achieved amazing things, I don't for a minute believe it couldn't have been done while also sparing the employee burnout, illness, and demoralization that are direct results of attempts to manipulate and control people's behavior by purposely inflicting stress.

This also goes for parents who believe they need to yell at their children to get results. One of the rules I teach in parenting classes is this: do not use anger as your primary method of behavioral control. I know children will "hop to" at times, and parents can get short-term behavioral compliance by using anger. But as with the angry CEO, this is a temporary fix, at best. At worst, directing anger at children repeatedly will put them into a chronic state of activation, and the accompanying inflammation will create avoidance patterns directed not only at parents, but also to the activities connected to the yelling, and other situational factors. By now I don't have to remind you how the long-term consequences of your stress switch constantly flipping on, no matter what the reason, can be devastating to an individual.

The expectation that "when I yell I get what I want" seems more and more pervasive in our society, especially with the easy accessibility of the internet to air our grievances. Social media and consumer reviews online can be used to threaten and punish businesses when someone doesn't get their way. Fear of this kind of retaliation creates over-reactivity on both sides that can create situations like the one I stumbled into at that Airbnb. This problem has gotten to the point where the hospitality industry is well known for quickly offering up freebies if people complain—a knee-jerk reaction intended to quiet the complainers (no matter how justified the complaint). It has become akin to giving a screaming baby a pacifier, and it's easy to see how it fosters a sense of personal entitlement.

Consumers know, too, that a minor inconvenience at a restaurant or hotel can turn into a free prize if they raise a big- and public-enough stink about it. Whole industries have allowed the fear of retaliation to activate their stress switches to incentivize a form of negative behavioral control over others, and in doing so, perpetuated a cycle of using stress to manipulate others. If we look at the chain reaction of stress this kind of behavioral control creates, it's not worth it. No amount of free stuff is worth contributing to the already rampant public health epidemic of stress. If we can change our thinking to give each other and ourselves some grace, instead of being perpetually caught up in judgment and entitlement, we'll all be better off for it. We don't need to dim another person's light to elevate and be brighter lights ourselves.

Lighthouses

At another, less stressful Airbnb during our real estate transition, my family found itself surrounded by lighthouses. The sweet woman who owned our rental had decorated it from wall to wall in lighthouses—yes, lighthouses in Arizona. I instantly loved it because of the parallels between lighthouses and life.

At one time in history, lighthouse lights used coal, which generated a great deal of soot. Lighthouse keepers spent most of their days removing the buildup of soot from the glass lenses. Today coal soot is not an issue, but lighthouse keepers still spend hours and hours every day diligently polishing, shining, and caring for their lights with such precision and effort. They know that if the light dims, or God forbid burns out, ships are going to wreck. It's important that the light be burning all the time.

We're all the keepers of our own lighthouses, responsible for tending to our own lights and preventing wrecks. The soot on our lenses is the buildup of all our traumatic experiences, stress, and triggers—all the things that need to be cleared away to live our best lives. If we continue letting it build up without wiping it away, the light inside will dim, eventually becoming invisible. The knowledge in this book can empower you to not only clear the soot that stress has built up for you in the past, but also to reduce the amount that occurs in the future. You'll have more time and energy for joy, leisure, love, and enrichment. We can choose to do the work to shine brightly and show others the way, or we can dim our guiding lights, leaving ourselves and others to flounder, lost in the darkness.

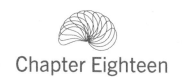

Chapter Eighteen

THE UNITED STATES OF STRESS

Especially with the new strategies and tools presented here, we each have the power to stabilize our own stress and make the conscious decision not to collude with other people's stress. But what about removing stress on a larger scale? What can be done for entire communities, nations, the world?

Imagine an impoverished village in a developing country with spiking levels of miscarriages in the pregnant women, rising levels of disease, and mortality trends on a worrying slope. To get to the bottom of what is happening in the village, we might start by looking at the stress factors affecting the larger community, examining the patterns of stress symptoms, and then, ripple by ripple, make our way inward to find a common cause for the community's several problems.

We might soon find that, because of the stress of poverty and overall living conditions in the village, many of the men have extremely reactive nervous states and are acting out in fight-or-flight stress, often violently, particularly towards the women and children. The constant presence of these live wires could easily create a cascading negative impact on the health of the other villagers.

This story is not imaginary, and unfortunately it plays out all too frequently in many developing countries, where entire populations of people are dealing not only with the ongoing survival fear, and hyper-vigilance brought on by poverty, but also all the catastrophic public health consequences of chronic stress. This is tragic, but we now understand clearly the cause-effect-cause cycle that is at work. Changing the paradigm on stress means using our better understanding to create better answers for the problems it causes.

I encountered this exact scenario consulting with a humanitarian team in Africa. A team I worked with came up with one strategy that has served to improve the current wellbeing of the village and will extend to future generations. The team proposed that moving the overly stressed and reactive men to a work site away from the village during the day would allow the women and children to achieve some level of homeostatic regulation for the bulk of the day. When implemented, this plan created a valuable reprieve from the constant drama and violence created by the men's overactive stress switches, and the resulting behavioral fallout began to subside.

If you think the cycle of poverty and violence is only happening in third world countries, please think again. There is a *huge* problem of violence that has embedded itself into our culture here in the United States. People hurt each other, and when you look at the cascade of events that has led someone to do violent harm to someone else, the stress switch is almost always the culprit.

Every person's stress has a ripple effect that touches everyone they have contact with, and it also touches the people those people have contact with, and so on. If you apply the idea of six degrees of separation, you can imagine the far-reaching impact one person's chronically active stress switch can have. Your stress simply is not just your stress—it is a virus you are willfully choosing to host, incubate, and then release into the world around you in varying doses. With better awareness—and now you have that awareness—you have not only the option but the responsibility to do something about your stress. When you take control of your stress switch, regulate your nervous system, and model the effects of being calm and untriggered for other people, you are actively choosing to make the world a better place.

I've seen it time and time again in my clinics—if you change one person's ability to regulate their stress, the ripple effect is set in motion, touching their family, friends, and everyone else they know. If enough people do this as a group the impact can spread throughout classrooms, workplaces, and entire communities. On the global level, the possibilities are truly endless. When we move away from a stress state, we move toward humanity and empathy for one another.

Humanity

My boyfriend and I had just arrived in Hawaii for a long overdue vacation when I was in a scary accident that left me with a head injury and potentially a damaged spine. While my boyfriend followed the ambulance to the hospital in his own car, I was strapped to a backboard for the forty-five minute long ambulance ride to the hospital. The pain and stress of the journey was excruciating, especially without my boyfriend at my side to comfort me. His trip took even longer, so I was alone not only in the ambulance but then for those most stressful first moments in the ER.

By the time we arrived, my body was flooded with adrenaline from fight-or-flight and my stress switch was in overdrive. I looked up desperately from my backboard at the intake nurse standing above me, clicking away on her computer. Due to the nature of our modern medical system, she was more focused on her documentation than on her patient, but I needed human compassion and connection more than anything in the world at that moment. She stopped at one point and looked down at me, and I felt a glimmer of hope, before seeing that she was holding out a clipboard with a form for me to sign. I felt like a number, not a human being, and the fact that my stress switch was turned on—and high—made all of it one hundred times worse. I began to panic.

Then, a miracle. My boyfriend walked in, immediately came to my side, gripped my hand tightly, and said, "Everything's okay. Don't worry about the trip. I'm here. Honey, if we need to spend the entire vacation in this room we'll still have a great time." Then he said something funny—I don't recall what it was—and my stress switch instantly eased off. I calmed down. In that spontaneous moment his compassion, physical touch, love, and humor obliterated my stress and I felt all was going to be OK.

At the end of the day, there's no substitute for human connection, and while we all have the power to give it to one another, it only comes from a place of calm. If your stress switch is on, it hinders your ability to connect.

If my boyfriend had come barging into that ER activated by his own stress, freaking out about my injuries and yelling at the nurse about paperwork, that would have been a completely different experience for me. I would have only been more triggered, potentially even compounding my injuries by inflaming my body even more.

Think about how many people do this in stressful situations, especially medical ones. Stressed out fathers-to-be and other family members create stress for expectant women trying to deliver new life into this world. The physical stress response literally blocks things that need to happen in the mother's body during the birthing process, and can even harm mother and baby. Maybe there was a good reason to sequester everyone away from the birthing woman except professional helpers like doulas, midwives, and doctors!

There is also research suggesting that the most extreme levels of traumatic stress—such as the Holocaust, war, or systemic poverty—can actually embed themselves in a person's DNA and cause problems in future generations. This is just another compelling piece of evidence that stress does not operate in a vacuum; that cruelty has an even larger and longer-lasting effect than we may think.

But the flip side of this implication is that humanity's capacity for love can also reach far beyond our understanding. We must focus on that—on shifting the conversation to love, kindness, and humanity. We must transcend the negatives of the stress epidemic, and embrace and nurture the positive. Then, we can live in a better world.

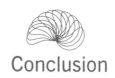

Conclusion

RISKING EVERYTHING

The medical community took more than ten years to accept that bacteria are the cause of peptic ulcers. Scientific data was mounting, and yet the medical establishment refused to believe it. At one point, one of those future Nobel-laureate researchers even sent a camera down to record his own ulcer-free GI tract. Then, he injected himself with the bacteria in question, sent the camera down again, and produced video evidence that he had now, in fact, developed brand-new ulcers. Then he treated his ulcers with an antibiotic, sent a camera down a third time, and the ulcers were gone. To reiterate—**he produced conclusive scientific evidence, and still the medical community refused to believe him.** They stubbornly folded their arms, pouted, and protested, "No! We won't believe that bacteria causes ulcers."

Why did they unreasonably and recklessly reject logical truth? Perhaps they were wary because Drs. Warren and Marshall received funding for their study from the pharmaceutical company that owned the patents for the antibiotic. However, it is clear that Warren and Marshall's study produced an empirically effective cure for disease. I would argue that the medical community collectively allowed emotional reasoning and a resistance to change to blind them. It is fine—and wise—to consider who has financial incentives to prove a new idea will work. However, it is worse than unwise to refuse a groundbreaking cure just because someone is promoting it.

The same could be said about me. Because one piece of my solution for stress happens to be a product I invented (TouchPoints), my credibility is a tempting target for a portion of the medical community. The million-dollar stress management industry would like everyone to ignore extensive, peer-reviewed, published research on the causes and successful treatment of stress.[45] They dumb their assessment down to this: "We won't believe her because she has a product." Apparently, in my case, suddenly science, inventions, and medical entrepreneurialism cannot be allowed to co-exist. Nevermind that every medical treatment we trust today was once a brand new discovery, or that TouchPoints are an *award-winning* product that has been shown over and over again to work. Since they were introduced, the TouchPoints devices have received the 2018 Edison Awards Gold Medal for Wellness Technology and several other international awards, have been featured by the Huffington Post and NBC News, and were named the Top Health and Wellness Tech at the 2019 Consumer Electronics Show by both *Forbes* and *Digital Trends* magazines.

I'm going to put a basic question to you: if there is clear evidence that something is safe, and it works—it works really well, in fact— would you be interested in it? Or would you be like the people who put their hands over their ears like children who aren't getting their way? And here's a more inciting question: what would you risk to see all the problems outlined in this book melt out of your life? Now, what would you do if, actually, you didn't have to risk all that at all?

The fact is, the bilateral stimulation technology in TouchPoints has been used safely for years, but was previously only available in a less-effective form via specialized medical devices, and only available in a doctor's or therapists' offices. Used in conjunction with EMDR therapy, it is a well-established standard treatment for PTSD.[46] Now, with an improved waveform, for the cost of one private therapy session (at the time of this book writing), people anytime and anywhere can use bilateral stimulation by wearing TouchPoints on their wrists like a wristwatch, or hiding them in pockets or socks. As a care and treatment provider, it's exciting to see the ways that having this treatment available in the moment of stress—not only days or weeks later during an office appointment—can contribute to faster healing and recovery.

I believe there is good cause for frustration here, but it is a mistake to take aim at scientists and inventors who are seeking new solutions. Instead I challenge all of us to protest the system that has failed to acknowledge progress and instead led people to believe that the options for chronic stress, PTSD, autism, ADHD, depression, and other disorders are only the same old treatments, and only available at a high price tag in their offices. The information about better options is available to them, and it is available to you!

The good news is that at the time I'm writing this, TouchPoints are being adopted globally by therapists, doctors, and individuals who want their well-documented results: relief from the sleep difficulties, irritation, and performance issues caused by stress. People are afraid of change, but despite the detractors, we are making waves and a movement is forming.

In all fairness, I was well aware of exactly what I was getting into from day one. In fact, when we first partnered, I warned our CEO, Vicki Mayo, that the stakes were high: "You realize I am risking professional annihilation with this," I said. "I've seen how these things unfold in the medical community." Yes, I knew I was making myself a target—but I am willing to risk it all, because I need to get this cure for stress into people's hands. I know it works. I'm willing because it's worth it.

Anyone tempted to question my motives can also consider that I've put my life savings into TouchPoints, and to date, I have not made one penny of it back. If I'm a "snake-oil salesman," I will tell you—I am a really bad one! TouchPoints are catching on, and I know the movement will grow—but this is not really about the money.

It is about me taking personal triumph in my own life and handing the hard-won treasure over to you. I know how to remove the mercury from our pond, and I am doing everything I can to make sure that that happens. Ironically, due to my own health story and life circumstances, I needed my invention more than I ever thought that I would in my lifetime. This is about having compassion and empathy for each individual that has walked in those shoes, suffering so much and for so long, and believing there was no light at the end of the tunnel.

This is about me standing up as a member of humanity, of the global community, and saying: here. I have a way to help. Try it before you deny it. I made these for you because I understand how bad it is to suffer from stress and all its satellite effects that wreck life as you know it and the lives of your loved ones around you. Once the mercury is in the pond, the clock is ticking. With every minute that passes, another piece of you is chipped away and falls into the abyss. Please let me help you because it's the best I can do. I don't know you, but I love you so much. You're so important to this world that I have literally risked everything in order to bring this solution to you. And that risk is one hundred percent worth it for me.

For more information, please visit www.amyserin.com.

NOTES

¹ "APA Stress Survey: Children Are More Stressed Than Parents Realize." *PracticeUpdate* vol. 6, no. 11 (APA Services, 2009), https://www.apaservices.org/practice/update/2009/11-23/stress-survey.

² "How Stress Influences Disease: Study Reveals Inflammation As the Culprit,"*Science Daily*, April 2, 2012, https://www.sciencedaily.com/releases/2012/04/120402162546.htm.

³ Angela Brownawell, "APA Survey Raises Concern About Parent Perceptions of Children's Stress," press release, *American Psychological Association,* November 3, 2009, https://www.apa.org/news/press/releases/2009/11/stress, (accessed April 10, 2019).

⁴ V. Menon, "Salience Network," in *Brain Mapping: An Encyclopedic Reference,* ed. Arthur W. Toga (Elsevier Academic Press, 2015), 597-611.

⁵ This is an oversimplified summary of Descartes' theory of dualism, but it reflects his core idea.

⁶ Susan Scutti, "One in Six US Adults Takes Psychiatric Drugs, Study Says," *CNN Online*, December 12, 2016, https://www.cnn.com/2016/12/12/health/psychiatric-drug-use/index.html (accessed April 4, 2019).

⁷ B. L. Smith, "Inappropriate prescribing," *Monitor on Psychology*, Vol. 43, No. 6 (2012): 36.

⁸ Ibid., 36.

⁹ A. Delfanti, "Tweaking Genes in Your Garage: Biohacking Between Activism and Entrepreneurship," in *Activist Media and Biopolitics: Critical Media Interventions in the Age of Biopower,* eds. W. Sützland and T. Hug (Innsbruck, Austria: Innsbruck University Press, 2012): 163-178.

¹⁰ For a good overall review of the correlation between supplement use and the incidence of cancer, see https://sciencebasedmedicine.org/vitamins-and-cancer-risk/.

¹¹ A. Serin, N.S. Hageman, and E. Kade, "The Therapeutic Effect of Bilateral Alternating Stimulation Tactile Form Technology on the Stress Response," *Journal of Biotechnology and Biomedical Science*, 1(2) (2018): 42.

¹² B.D. Perry and others. "Childhood Trauma, the Neurobiology of Adaptation, and "Use-dependent" Development of the Brain: How "States" Become "Traits," *Infant Mental Health Journal vol. 16, no. 4* (1995): 271-291.

¹³ R. B. McCall, "The Development of Intellectual Functioning in Infancy and the Prediction of Later IQ," in *Handbook of Infant Development*, ed. J.D. Osofsky (Wiley: New York, 1979).

¹⁴ J. N. McCall, "Research on the Psychological Effects of Orphanage Care: A Critical Review," in *Rethinking Orphanages for the 21st Century.* ed. R.B. McKenzie (Sage: Newbury Park, CA, 1999).

[15] The St. Petersburg-USA Orphanage Research Team, "The Effects of Early Social-emotional and Relationship Experience on the Development of Young Orphanage Children," *Monographs of the Society for Research in Child Development*, 73(3) (2008), http://doi.org/10.1111/j.1540-5834.2008.00483.x

[16] H. Larkin, J.J. Shields, and R.F. Anda, "The Health and Social Consequences of Adverse Childhood Experiences (ACES) Across the Lifespan: an Introduction to Prevention and Intervention in the Community," *Journal of Prevention and Intervention in the Community*, 40(4) (2012): 263-70.

[17] Vincent J Felitti and others, "Relationship of Childhood Abuse and Household Dysfunction to Many of the Leading Causes of Death in Adults," *American Journal of Preventive Medicine*, 14(4) (1998): 245-258.

[18] To learn more, visit the Center for Disease Control's ACE Study website at https://www.cdc.gov/violenceprevention/childabuseandneglect/acestudy/index.html.

[19] R. F. Anda and others. "The Enduring Effects of Abuse and Related Adverse Experiences in Childhood: A Convergence of Evidence from Neurobiology and Epidemiology," *European Archives of Psychiatry and Clinical Neuroscience*, 256(3) (2006): 174–186. http://doi.org/10.1007/s00406-005-0624-4.

[20] A. Danese, and others. "Adverse Childhood Experiences and Adult Risk Factors for Age-related Disease, Depression, Inflammation, and Clustering of Metabolic Risk Markers," *Archives of Pediatric and Adolescent Medicine*, 163(12) (2009): 1135–1143. http://doi.org/10.1001/archpediatrics.2009.214

[21] B. S. McEwen, "Allostasis and Allostatic Load: Implications for Neuropsychopharmacology," *Neuropsychopharmacology*, 22(2) (2000): 108-124.

[22] In 2013, the WHO released new recommended protocols for mental health care after trauma, and specifically highlighted these two therapies as effective. For more information, visit: https://www.who.int/mediacentre/news/releases/2013/trauma_mental_health_20130806/en/

[23] This is not the same thing as electroconvulsive therapy, which is a severe kind of therapy for extreme cases. CES involves a very small electrical current and it doesn't cause brain damage. Many people consider it to be non-invasive, and it is FDA approved for anxiety, insomnia, and depression.)

[24] L. H. Trahan, and others. "The Flynn Effect: A Meta-analysis," *Psychological Bulletin*, 140(5) (2014): 1332.

[25] G. D. Farmer, S. Baron-Cohen, and W. J. Skylark, "People with Autism Spectrum Conditions Make More Consistent Decisions," *Psychological Science*, 28(8) (2017): 1067-1076.

[26] For a good review of common cognitive distortions, visit: https://psychcentral.com/lib/15-common-cognitive-distortions/

[27] For more information, see: http://cogprints.org/677/1/ulcers.htm

[28] C. Hadley, "The Infection Connection: Helicobacter Pylori Is More Than Just the Cause of Gastric Ulcers—It Offers An Unprecedented Opportunity to Study Changes in Human Microecology and the Nature of Chronic Disease," *EMBO Reports*, 7(5) (2006): 470–473. http://doi.org/10.1038/sj.embor.7400699

[29] T. L. Testerman, and J. Morris, "Beyond the Stomach: An Updated View of Helicobacter pylori Pathogenesis, Diagnosis, and Treatment" *World Journal of Gastroenterology*, 20(36) (2014): 12781–12808. http://doi.org/10.3748/wjg.v20.i36.12781

[30] Daniel Trotta, "Patriots QB Tom Brady After Super Bowl Loss: 'I Expect to Be Back," *Huffpost Online*, February 5, 2018, https://www.huffington post.com/entry/super-bowl-tom-brady_us_5a7805dbe4b06ee97af47972 (accessed April 4, 2019).

[31] K. H. Teigen, "Yerkes-Dodson: A Law for All Seasons," *Theory & Psychology*, 4(4) (1994): 525-547.

[32] E. F. Loftus and J. E. Pickrell, "The Formation of False Memories" *Psychiatric Annals*, 25(12) (1995): 720-725. https://blogs.brown.edu/recoveredmemory/files/2015/05/Loftus_Pickrell_PA_95.pdf

[33] R. M. Kramer, "Revisiting the Bay of Pigs and Vietnam Decisions 25 Years Later: How Well Has the Groupthink Hypothesis Stood the Test of Time?" *Organizational Behavior and Human Decision Processes*, 73(2-3) (1998): 236-271. http://dx.doi.org/10.1006/obhd.1998.2276 2

[34] Incidentally, if Darwin were alive today, the recent advances in neuroscience would no doubt astonish him, especially the ones I'm talking about throughout this book, all of which could have altered the outcome of his experiment.

[35] You can find the Holmes-Rahe Stress Inventory online at: https://www.stress.org/holmes-rahe-stress-inventory/

[36] A. Keller, and others. "Does the Perception That Stress Affects Health Matter? The Association with Health and Mortality." *Health Psychology: Official Journal of the Division of Health Psychology*, American Psychological Association, 31(5)   (2011):   677-84. https://www.ncbi.nlm.nih.gov/pmc/articles/PMC3374921/

[37] D. Danner, and others. "Positive Emotions in Early Life and Longevity" *Journal of Personality and Social Psychology*, 80(5) (2001): 804-813. www.apa.org/pubs/journals/releases/psp805804.pdf

[38] In the TouchPoint Challenge, you and/or your therapist stimulates a stressful event while you are wearing the devices so you can quickly feel—and measure—the stress reduction. For more information about TouchPoints and the Challenge, visit www.touchpoints.com.

[39] Dr. Michael Breus, widely known as "The Sleep Doctor," is an acknowledged sleep expert and regularly appears in national media sharing his expertise. You can find the glasses and more about them at https://thesleepdoctor.com/2018/12/17/christmas-gift-guide-for-the-best-sleep-products-of-2018/.

[40] Definitions and diagnostic criteria for the varying symptoms and manifestations of chronic, traumatic, and acute stress are still shifting within the mental health industry. The use of the terms post-traumatic stress disorder, complex post-traumatic stress disorder, acute stress disorder, and many others are often debated among researchers and other professionals. My purpose here is not to engage in those debates but to help you become more aware and informed. Please seek professional assistance for specific information and treatment if you think you might need help.

[41] R. Sinha, "Chronic Stress, Drug Use, and Vulnerability to Addiction," *Annals of the New York Academy of Sciences*, 1141(1) (2008): 105–130. https://www.ncbi.nlm.nih.gov/pmc/articles/PMC2732004/#

[42] You can learn more about the Trauma Recovery/HAP® organization and their work at www.emdrhap.org.

[43] Konuk, and others. "The Effects of Eye Movement Desensitization and Reprocessing (EMDR) therapy on Posttraumatic Stress Disorder in Survivors of the 1999 Marmara, Turkey, Earthquake" *International Journal of Stress Management*, 13 (3) (2006): 291.

[44] Ruth Umoh, "Steve Jobs to PepsiCo's Indra Nooyi: Don't be Too Nice," *CNBC Online*, August 6, 2018, https://www.cnbc.com/2018/08/06/3-things-pepsico-ceo-indra-nooyi-learned-from-apple-founder-steve-jobs.html (accessed April 4, 2019).

[45] For a selected peer-reviewed bibliography of my own research on stress as well as research specifically on TouchPoints, I invite you to visit https://serincenter.com.

[46] T. Amano and M. Toichi, "The Role of Alternating Bilateral Stimulation in Establishing Positive Cognition" in *EMDR therapy: A Multi-Channel Near-Infrared Spectroscopy Study* (2016). *PloS one*, 11(10), e0162735. doi:10.1371/journal.pone.0162735.